SMILE!

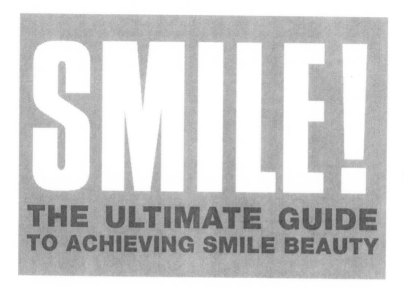

SMILE!

THE ULTIMATE GUIDE
TO ACHIEVING SMILE BEAUTY

JONATHAN B. LEVINE, DMD,

founder of GoSMILE

WITH JANE LARKWORTHY

WITH A FOREWORD BY MARISKA HARGITAY

WARNER
WELLNESS

NEW YORK   BOSTON

The information herein in not intended to replace the services of trained health professionals. You are advised to consult with your health care professional with regard to matters relating to your health, and in particular regarding matters that may require diagnosis or medical attention.

Copyright © 2006 by Jonathan B. Levine, DMD
All rights reserved.

Foreword copyright © 2006 by Mariska Hargitay
Warner Wellness

Warner Books
Time Warner Book Group
1271 Avenue of the Americas, New York, NY 10020
Visit our Web site at www.twbookmark.com.

Warner Wellness and the Warner Wellness logo are trademarks of Time Warner Book Group, Inc.

Printed in the United States of America

First Edition: March 2006

Library of Congress Cataloging-in-Publication Data

Levine, Jonathan B.
   Smile! : the ultimate guide to achieving smile beauty / Jonathan B. Levine with Jane Larkworthy. — 1st ed.
      p. cm.
   Includes index.
   ISBN-13: 978-0-446-69247-8
   ISBN-10: 0-446-69427-4
   1. Dentistry—Aesthetic aspects. 2. Beauty, Personal. 3. Smile. 4. Face. I. Larkworthy, Jane. II. Title.
   RK54.L48 2006
   617.6'01—dc22

                                                      2005022642

Illustrations by Meredith Noyes
Book design by HRoberts Design

ACKNOWLEDGMENTS

From playing lacrosse at Cornell University to being the CEO/Chairman of GoSMILE, our luxury oral care company, for me, it has always been about the *who*: Who I was spending time with, who I was learning from, and who I was experiencing life with.

My journey has been about being the best I can be with the people I love and respect. From my earliest memories, my mom and dad taught me that in whatever I chose to do, with hard work, I would succeed. This work ethic has never left me. I am driven every day to achieve and to feel productive.

My lacrosse coach at Cornell, Richie Moran, taught me how to focus on being the best that I could possibly be. In my senior year, we won the National Championship—it was one of the most exciting days of my life. My teammates and I learned that with the right mix of passion, hard work, and respect for each other, we could achieve anything.

At Boston University School of Graduate Dentistry, the focus was on the highest level of learning in order to offer state-of-the-art thinking and technical excellence to our future patients. This was ingrained in us by the leaders of the school, who were also leaders in their field: Gerald Kramer in periodontics, Herb Schilder in endodontics, Spencer Frankl as dean, Tom Kilgore in oral surgery, Val Wells, and John McManama in restorative dentistry.

Once out of dental school, I moved to New York City to start working. There, in 1981, I met a talented young ceramist, Adrian Jurim, who was working on a new technique called porcelain veneers. With Adrian's help, I eventually became one of the first dentists in the country to apply porcelain veneers and began lecturing about dental aesthetics.

After practicing dentistry for five years, I felt that I wanted to continue my education and specialize in prosthodontics, which focuses on aesthetics and reconstructive dentistry. My mentors during that time, in particular, were Dennis Tarnow and Harold Litvack—both amazing dentists.

Once I got out of the program in 1989, I opened my practice in New York City. With the help of lectures and learnings from Peter Dawson, DDS, of the Pankey Institute in Florida, and meetings at the Academy of Aesthetics, I developed my skills as a prosthodontist with a strong focus on aesthetics.

Today, twenty years later, through experiences with my patients, my technicians, and my colleagues, I have developed a very personalized way of creating beautiful smiles for people. I take a collaborative approach in understanding the needs and wants of my patients to deliver smiles that harmonize with their faces. My goal is to give people their most beautiful smiles possible. I love my work week, which is split between my clinical practice, my teaching position as educational director of the Aesthetics Program in the Continuing Education Department of NYU, and of course, my involvement with GoSMILE. Each effort positively reinforces the others, and I feel blessed to be surrounded by the most incredible people in each of these areas. At GoSMILE we are creating innovative products that can impact many people and help them to have a healthy, beautiful smile. We are involved with a wonderful organization called Operation Smile. The people at Operation Smile change the lives of young children all over the world born with cleft lip, cleft palate, and craniofacial defects. It's amazing to see how a 45-minute operation can change someone's life forever. The smile is so awesome, it makes us feel so good to give one and so great to receive one.

This book was a collaborative effort among many. Thanks to: Meredith Noyes for her unique Smile Beauty illustrations; to Samantha Ettus for being my friend and supporter, who gave me the confidence to do this book; to Diana Baroni for her terrific help; to my assistants, Kate Gibson and Enis Guri; to Mariska Hargitay for her generous soul and her beautiful smile; to my co-author, Jane Larkworthy, who made writing this book with her pure fun—I will miss our Sunday mornings; to my team of professionals in my aesthetic dental practice; and to my team of rock stars who comprise GoSMILE, especially my friend and partner Josh Shaw who is an inspiration every day; to my boys Cody and Julian; to my beautiful wife, Stacey, who wakes up every single day with a smile and the inner passion to make it all worthwhile; and to my mom who taught me that learning is a life process—this book is dedicated to her.

CONTENTS

FOREWORD

have a picture of myself as a child, posing in a family portrait. Everyone's face is more or less serious, but there I am on the end, smiling from ear to ear. I love that picture, and I love that smile: it's like a summary of everything I wanted to say to the world.

When I see someone smile, I am at ease. I am delighted, interested, charmed, and intrigued. I trust where it comes from, and I like what it says. In this book, Jonathan Levine celebrates the importance of a great smile and tells readers how they can improve theirs. Readers can benefit—inside and out—from the advice offered here.

I saw a TV makeover show once where a girl was struggling with her physical appearance. She had a whole list of procedures planned, but by far the most marked change in her came when she was given the gift of a perfect smile. And it wasn't perfect because it was stunningly beautiful; it was perfect because with it she was finally able to communicate who she was and who she wanted to be. It was almost as if she had suddenly learned a language everyone around her had spoken all her life, and now she too could join in the conversation. She cried big tears of joy when she looked in the mirror for the first time (I cried too), then smiled her gorgeous, generous smile.

Through this book, Jonathan Levine celebrates that woman, as I celebrate that little girl in my family portrait, both of us giving voice to what is within us, welcoming the world, asking the world to welcome us, and letting our smiles reflect our souls' delight.

—Mariska Hargitay

WHAT'S IN A SMILE?

Smiling: The art of speaking . . . without saying a word.

"Smile at life, and life will smile at you."
—William Shakespeare

There's a reason why the smile is the universal language. The original form of instant messaging, a smile is ageless and it never goes out of style.

In the past few years, the smile has taken center stage as the ultimate symbol of beauty—more than beautiful eyes, more than great hair, even more than a sexy body. A brilliant smile has become the determinant in describing both beauty and personality. Think about it: You never hear someone say, "She's got such a great smile," when they're describing an aloof or rude woman. Rather, such appraisal evokes admiration, even envy. She is someone you'd like to model yourself after.

A smile is one of the greatest gifts you can give somebody. Equally, it's one of the greatest gifts to receive. Wouldn't life be better if we all smiled more?

FACT

It takes nearly three times the number of muscles to frown as it does to smile. Frowning requires forty-three, while smiling asks only seventeen to help out. Stop working so hard!

Smiling is also one of the most natural movements a body makes. We were all born with the ability to smile. In the very first few weeks of infancy, babies automatically begin smiling on their own. Within two months, they're usually starting to recognize when others are smiling at them, and, by this time, they're reciprocating in kind. Who needs their baby to figure out how to roll over when he's tossing a fresh, innocent, gleeful smile back to you? Here's a sad statistic about growing up: Babies smile an average of two hundred times a day; the average woman smiles sixty-two times a day. The average man smiles only eight.

SMILING MAKES YOU BEAUTIFUL

Think of people whose smiles you admire. Watch how they tilt their head or engage their eyes a bit when they do it. These are not conscious additions; they are natural characteristics that come about individually when someone smiles. Smiles create other natural characteristics as well—beautiful ones that form from years of, well, happiness—like that little crinkle in the nose, the creases around the eyes, and the aptly named smile lines. These are part of a great natural smile; you should have them. Mark Twain put it best: "Wrinkles should merely indicate where smiles have been."

Scientific studies have shown that people actually respond more to the act of someone's smile than to how perfect or white that smile is. There is a message of affability in a smile. It says, "Feel free to approach me. I'm interested in what you have to say." There's a lost opportunity when you feel that your smile doesn't have those implications. You're missing out on great things, from meeting interesting people to the basic pleasures of enjoyment.

SMILING MAKES FRIENDS AND INFLUENCES PEOPLE

A strong smile has power. It increases the production of serotonin, which has been scientifically proven to elevate the mood of both the person giving the smile and the person receiving it. A full, genuine smile automatically exudes confidence. It's a widely held belief that people with great smiles are more self-assured. According to the Smarter Smile Survey (conducted by Harris Interactive for Align Technology, October 2000), 64 percent agree that people with nice smiles are more outgoing. Eighty-seven percent think that your smile is very important to your self-esteem. You can't ignore the general consensus. Every element of the smile is connected to confidence. Roughly six in ten adults believe that if they had a whiter smile, it would boost their self-confidence, according to a study sponsored by Orbit chewing gum. The study also found that 71 percent believe people with nice smiles make friends far more easily than those with crooked teeth.

The smile has a profound effect not only on our perception of someone's attractiveness, but on what we think about that person as well. A great smile is associated with good health and is sometimes even a barometer of wealth. Someone with noticeably flawed teeth is usually presumed to be suffering financially. In contrast, studies have shown that a white, aligned smile signals that someone is healthy, smart, and financially secure. You'll find evidence of this simply by digging up your high school or college yearbook. Check out the students with the big, confident grins. Studies have proven that students with the big, broad, and gleaming smiles are more likely to have had successful careers and solid marriages than their poker-faced peers.

"Facial expressions are critically important in all ways of how we communicate. It's what we see first, what we respond to first, and, right or wrong, it's what we base our first impressions on," says clinical psychologist Sylvia Welsh, PhD. "So if you have a warm smile, you're likely to evoke warmth in others. What you put out is what you get back. If you're uncomfortable with your smile, it will affect everything in your life. People won't respond to you as much as you'd like them to. You might even be inadvertently creating a hostile environment. Depression is something people actually try to stay away from, whereas happiness conveys something much more contagious."

A SMILE CAN MAKE YOU YOUNGER

Smiles are also associated with youth. So why do so many people attempt to forestall the aging process by suffering through face-lifts, chemical peels, and microliposuction when an aesthetic dentist can fix an aging smile?

Doing nothing more than readjusting what's inside your mouth can take ten years off your face.

As we age, our teeth shorten, creating dark silhouettes, which are referred to as negative space. By lengthening those teeth, they become visible again when you're speaking and even when your lips are in a relaxed smile position. This regained tooth exposure translates to a more youthful face overall. Another consequence of aging teeth is yellowing. An in-office whitening treatment and/or the right over-the-counter whitener can restore that youthful whiteness. New technology has made these kinds of problems very easy to fix, and many of my patients have forgone the knife, laser, and needle in favor of changing their smile.

TRANSFORM YOUR SMILE

Back in the 1950s, more than half of the adult population over the age of sixty-five had lost all of their natural teeth. This decade, only a third of that group is in the same predicament. In 1960, Americans over sixty-five had an average of only seven of their original teeth. Today that number has risen to an average of twenty-four.

It also wasn't so long ago that people who didn't have a flawed smile were the rare exception. As recently as the early 1990s, a flawless smile was expected only from movie stars and beauty queens.

But that's all changed. Somewhere in the past decade or two, the way a smile looks has become almost as important as how well it works. Sure, we rely on our teeth to perform their intended functions, such as helping us chew and speak, and supporting the face's structure. But function alone isn't enough anymore. If a smile is unevenly aligned or has a gray or yellow cast, it's not enough for most of us. A smile now needs to look as close to flawless as it can.

SETTING THE STAGE

Think of your smile as a stage set for a play. The lips are the curtains, and the front teeth are the main characters. As the lips part, the curtain is rising, and the actors should be in their proper position, set to give the stage balance and harmony. Whether your own dentist ever uses this analogy or not, he's thinking of the smile this way. He's thinking of how the lips move in comparison with the teeth. He's thinking of your two front teeth, the central incisors, as the stars and he examines how they're set up against the other supporting actors, your canines—looking to create a balance. It's all about the balance—of the set (your face and mouth), the actors (your teeth), and their placement.

DENTISTS AREN'T JUST CAVITY FILLERS ANYMORE

Dental offices aren't the dens of pain that we remember from our childhoods. Instead, dental practices today represent the opportunity for aesthetic improvement. Seventy-seven million baby boomers want to look and feel younger, and major dental care companies such as Procter & Gamble (who make Crest) and Colgate-Palmolive are spending millions on advertising tooth-whitening products and other technological advancements in cosmetic dentistry.

Smile nuisances can be fixed at any age, so you can

start feeling better about yours as soon as you put your mind to it. Once you feel better about your smile, you will, without question, use it more. And so begins the wonderful ripple effect: If you start smiling more, that person who you smiled at now smiles at someone else, and so on and so on. It's like that old Fabergé Organics commercial—tell two friends, and so on. It's a chain reaction. Smile at someone, and they can't help but smile back.

SMILE ASSESSMENT: GRADE YOUR SMILE

Find a mirror and take a look at your smile. If you don't love what you see, you're certainly not alone. In fact, only 50 percent of Americans are happy with their smiles. If you fall into that group, you'll get nowhere denying it—perhaps it's time to make a change.

This book is based on the premise that there is no reason not to love your smile. Your smile could be as magnetic as Julia Roberts's, as lovely as Halle Berry's, as alluring as Scarlett Johansson's. I don't know these actresses' dental histories, but most celebrities with world-famous grins weren't born with them. We're all human. And we're all entitled to enhance what we were born with.

STAY TRUE TO YOUR SMILE

Those celebrity smiles raise another pertinent issue. I can't stress enough how important it is to stay true to your own individual smile. Of course, it's only natural to want it whiter or straighter, but the farther you stray from the smile you were born with, the less your smile will look like it's actually yours. Think about all the bad plastic surgery you see on the street and television every day: The best work is on those who don't look like they've had anything done to them. Smiles are no exception. Dentistry needs to be invisible.

Take my patient Christie Brinkley. Hers is a hundred-watt model-perfect smile. Her teeth are beautifully aligned, and she's got those two sexy full central incisors leading the way. But put Christie's smile on, say, Natalie Portman and it wouldn't work. Just as people wave pages from magazines in their hairdresser's face demanding Meg's or Jennifer's hair, patients come to me every day begging for Julia's smile. But even imagining any of these celebrities' smiles on another celebrity illustrates how easy it is to miss the point. You shouldn't want someone else's smile. You should want yours, as good as it can be. It's up to you and your dental professional to attain it.

Now that the smile is quickly becoming the epicenter of beauty, we have begun to care as much now about having a dazzling one as we do about having our abs tight or our skin clear. And while those two latter attributes have always been up there on the list of vanity concerns, a fabulous smile has only recently risen up to the top of the list. Smiles are just one more reflection of vitality and youth.

With the myriad advancements in dental technology and the vast strides in home care and all that we know about successfully maintaining oral health, anyone can have a great smile.

This book isn't aimed to help you achieve Christie's or Julia's or Halle's or Tom's smile. It is written to guide you toward the smile you were meant to have. In here, you'll find the answers to every smile dilemma and the solutions to every smile problem. But most important, it will guide you to getting—and keeping—your own smile beauty.

ONE

FINDING THE RIGHT DENTIST FOR YOU

According to the Mintel consumer intelligence report on oral care, only 68 percent of Americans have visited their dentist in the past year and a half. That number continues to rise as health care benefits improve and patients learn more about both their teeth and the options in dentistry.

Going to the dentist should not be the anxiety-filled experience you may have had as a child, squeezing your eyes shut, gripping the chair with all your might, silently making a pact with God that you'd never eat candy again if just once they didn't find any cavities. You're not a kid anymore. You have a say in whether your dental appointment will be a positive or negative experience. Just follow the steps I've laid out, and both the anxiety—and the pain—will be taken out of the equation.

STEP ONE: SQUARE ONE

When it comes to your smile, that part of your body that wins friends and influences people, you don't want to offer it up to just any dentist. Whether you have recently moved and are not familiar with dentists in the area or are not completely satisfied with the care you are currently receiving, the following guidelines will help you find the right one for you.

- Ask for recommendations. Talk to people who've had the kind of dentistry you require. How do you know who to ask? That's easy. Ask anyone whose smile you admire. If they respond, "This is my natural smile!" compliment them, then move on to the next person. You're eventually going to hit someone whose natural-looking smile is *not* the smile they were born with.
- Call the prosthodontic department of your nearby university's graduate dental school (the prosthodontic department specializes in restorative dentistry and reconstruction of the mouth). Or, if there's an aesthetic program, ask the faculty who's on its recommendation list.
- Make sure the dentist recommended to you doesn't teach more than one to two days a week. A full-time dental academic would be the ideal professor, should you decide to study dentistry, but when it comes to dental work, you want one who's more involved in clinical practice.

- Contact the American Academy of Esthetic Dentistry (www.estheticacademy.org; 312-321-5121). This is a reputable organization whose members are an esteemed group of professionals.
- Do *not* call 800-DENTIST or 800-SMILE-GREAT or 800-*anything* teeth-related: Dentists pay to get on these phone lists. The only ones recommending them are themselves.

STEP TWO: NARROWING YOUR SEARCH

Once you get some dentists' names, call their offices and conduct a phone interview with each one. The first checkpoint for clearance depends on the answers they give you. Without exception, ask the following:

- "Does she work with different specialists?" If the receptionist replies, "Oh, she's extremely talented. She does the root canals, oral surgery, perio, even orthodontics," say, "No thank you," and move on to the next name on your list. No dental professional is good at every specialty. You want someone who works with a team of specialists to handle the different divisions of dentistry.
- "And can you tell me some of the names of the specialists she usually works with?" You should *absolutely* ask this question, then check on the specialists' names as well. Professional football players wouldn't

train with—or be in the same league with—a high school team. You get the analogy.

- "Does she have hygienists? Who's doing the cleaning? A hygienist or the dentist?" If the receptionist says that the dentist is doing the cleaning, say, "Thank you" again and hang up again. Cleaning is a hygienist's specialty.
- "How much time will a routine cleaning take?" It should last at least forty-five minutes.
- "Has Dr. So-and-So been published?" And by that, I don't mean before-and-after ads on the subway or a Web site with dancing molars. Ask if this dentist has been quoted in reputable magazines or whether any of his works have been published in a professional dental journal.
- "Does she give lectures? Where? How often?" The lectures should be at either a reputable dental school or the local university and should be as recent as within the past year.

STEP THREE: EVALUATING A VISIT

Upon your first visit to a new dentist, schedule a consultation only, with no dental work. Remember, you should be interviewing the dentist as much as the dentist is interviewing you. After all, this is a potential employee you'll be paying. Don't just ask questions, but observe the surroundings.

- **His best work:** Ask to see photographs of patients he's treated who've had similar conditions.

- **What's her specialty?** Ask if she's a dental specialist, such as a prosthodontist. (Does she do a lot of restorative dentistry?) If her answer is, "Oh, I do all kinds of dental specialties," head for the hills! A dentist cannot (and should not) do all things. If you're in a metropolitan area, especially, there should be a different specialist to go to for each area of dentistry.

- **Sterilized for your safety:** Is there a dedicated sterilization area? Ask the dentist: "Do you have an autoclave?"(An autoclave is a heat sterilizer. Every instrument that goes in the mouth should be autoclaved.) Check to see (or ask) whether all the examining rooms are barrier-controlled for full sterilization. You can tell by asking (or checking to see) whether everything used is covered with plastic.

- **In-house tech support:** Ask which technicians he works with (ceramist, metal technician), and for how long. The best answer is: "We have an in-house lab." And the longer he's been working with this technician, the better.

Further, you know you're really in a top-notch practice if there are on-site laboratories with ceramists (a ceramist is the person who makes the porcelain veneers), plaster technicians (they prepare the mouth model for the ceramist), and metal technicians (they create the substructures for the bridges and implant crowns). Any lab with lab technicians will have the latest ceramic equipment.

While having every piece of state-of-the-art equipment does not necessarily guarantee expert care, the following technologies can help your dentist provide the high-quality care you are seeing. Ask if the practice uses any of the following:

- Digital X-rays.
- Digital cameras.
- The latest autoclave equipment.
- Fiber-optic hand pieces.
- Magnification eyeglasses for the dentist.

You should also inquire about patient communication technology, which can aid your dentist in explaining whatever concerns she may have or procedures she may propose. Ask if she uses:

- Computer imaging.
- Patient education software.
- Intra-oral camera.

Finally, don't underestimate the value of office aesthetics. Make sure to ask yourself: Do the office, examining rooms, staff, and environment seem dedicated to making patients comfortable?

SPECIAL MEDICAL CONCERNS: WHAT TO KNOW BEFORE YOU GO

Before you get in the dentist's chair, reviewing this list will help prevent potential bumps later on.

Bleeding

- If you bleed easily, check with your physician as to whether this could influence your dental appointment.
- Heart conditions may require medication, such as Coumadin, which thins the blood and can therefore cause an increase in bleeding.

Heart-Related Issues

- If you have any heart-related issues (mitral valve prolapse, heart murmurs, congenital heart defects), find out from your cardiologist whether you have regurgitation or not. If you do, you need to be premedicated one hour before getting dental work.
- Heart conditions and structural defects also increase the risk of developing a heart valve infection called endocarditis after dental procedures. Bacterial endocarditis can occur when bacteria travel through the bloodstream to the heart and colonize there. Bacteria circulate in the bloodstream and should flow through smoothly when they reach the heart. But any heart abnormalities can potentially cause

bacteria to cling on and ignite infection. This is why antibiotics are given to patients with heart conditions before dental procedures with high bleeding potential (extractions, root canals, scaling and root planing, implant placements, even standard cleaning on certain bleeding-prone patients)—it's done to stave off infection.

Sensitivities or Allergies to Medications

- If you're allergic to penicillin, novocaine, or any other medications, always be sure to tell your dentist or hygienist.
- If you're allergic to an oral antibiotic, your dentist will most likely instruct you to take an alternative that you are not allergic to.
- If you're taking *any* type of medication, always be sure to tell your dentist or hygienist.

Pregnancy

- If there is any chance that you are pregnant, or you know you are, it's advisable to avoid major dental procedures whenever possible. However, in the event that dental work can't wait, the only anesthetic used should be Carbocaine. Unlike local anesthetics, such as Xylocaine or Septocaine (updated brand names for the now antiquated novocaine), Carbocaine contains no epinephrine (a synthetic adrenaline), which can put the fetus at potential risk.

- As most are aware, pregnant and potentially pregnant women should not be x-rayed. But once again, on the rare occasion when an X-ray can't wait, make sure that it's a digital X-ray and that two aprons are placed over you.

- One thing that many people don't know, however, is that hormonal changes brought on by pregnancy render gums more susceptible to plaque. Thus, if you are pregnant, you should get dental cleanings more often.

FAMILY VALUES

When should your child's first dental appointment be? Once teeth begin to appear, you should start thinking about scheduling your child's first dental appointment. Most dentists recommend the first visit around age three, or earlier if you notice any staining or have other concerns.

- **Prep yourself:** Call your dentist and ask him to explain to you what goes on during a child's first visit, so you can then prepare your child for what to expect. Also, be sure to bring your child's medical history with you to the appointment.

- **Prep your child:** Instead of instilling fear in your child about the dentist, get her excited about doing something as grown-up as going for a checkup. Explain how important it is for people to take care of their teeth. Explain the procedures she will encounter, such as the big reclining chair and the bib, the big light that looks like a smile, and the cool probing mouth mirror. Reading together a child's book about going to the dentist will help get your child excited and also waylay any fears of this unfamiliar visit. A couple of good books are *My Dentist Makes Me Smile* by Leslie Craig (1stBooks Library) and *Open Wide! A Visit to the Dentist* by Cecile Schoberle (Simon Spotlight/Nickelodeon).

The first visit is more of an introductory one, where the child is shown around, so to speak, checking out the sights (the big illuminating light, the swinging X-ray machine) and sounds (the suction tube, the electric toothbrush—the drill can be saved for later) to help familiarize him with the dentist's office. Instead of a fear zone, the dentist's office can be one of wonder—it's up to you as the parent to set the example. If your dentist wants to spend some time alone with your child, that's fine (if your child seems comfortable). It's important for the dentist to establish a relationship and trust with your child. Once a child is comfortable in the dentist's office, the visit should last about twenty to thirty minutes. The visit may include the following, depending on the child's age:

- An examination of the teeth, bite, gums, and oral tissues to monitor growth and development.
- A discussion among the three of you on proper at-home oral care.

- A possible discussion about fluoride needs.
- Nutritional advice for healthy teeth.
- A gentle tooth polishing, which can be an exciting and positive way to end a first visit (the whirring of the brush, the grape flavor of the toothpaste, the smooth feeling of teeth afterward).

TWO

THE ELEMENTS OF A SUCCESSFUL DENTAL VISIT

THE CLEANING

Any problems your smile has, or any nascent difficulties, will be caught early by your hygienist. Get a professional cleaning from your hygienist two to three times a year, more often if you've had a sizable amount of dental work done. She'll find the plaque that you've missed, she'll scrape off the tartar that your brush and floss can't, and in doing this she'll help keep cavities and other complications away. Professional cleanings are like insurance for your smile. The investment can save you thousands of dollars in the long run, as smaller problems diagnosed along the way can prevent much bigger ones from occurring later on.

The purpose of a professional cleaning is not only to remove the tartar above the gum and bacterial-induced deposits below the gum, as well as to polish off extrinsic stains from teeth, but also to get a comprehensive lesson in oral care. As she goes through each step of the cleaning process, your hygienist should explain what she's doing, why she's doing it, and why your teeth may be sensitive or may start bleeding. An adjustable mirror or an intra-oral camera (a more high-tech version of the mirror) is attached to the examining light, which allows patients to watch her at work and understand what she's talking about. It's one thing to hear your hygienist say, "You really need to pay more attention to your back molars." But it's quite another thing to actually see her working on those back molars and fully comprehend what that work involves so you can replicate it at home. Finally, based on the condition she finds your mouth in, she should give you an updated primer on the certain oral care techniques you need to incorporate into your home care routine.

BE NOT AFRAID

With the availability of topical anesthetics, even a challenging cleaning should not hurt. If you find that you're wincing every thirty seconds or so, or you are bleeding more than a little, the dental hygienist may be cleaning too aggressively. It's likely she's going too deep and removing your inner epithelium (the inner lining

CLEANING IS NOT A DENTIST'S JOB

Cleaning is the hygienist's area of expertise. She went to school for this; she's been trained for this. This allows your dentist to concentrate on his own areas of expertise. This arrangement makes for a better, more productive environment—it's a healthy check-and-balance system. Even the dentist who's starting out and struggling to get his practice on its feet should still have his own hygienist.

of the gum that rests on the tooth) inadvertently. The best way to address the problem is by addressing the hygienist directly. Stop her and ask, "Why is this hurting so much?" "Are my gums inflamed?" Topical anesthetics are usually applied to ease any pain or discomfort.

THE CAVITY, AND THE VARIOUS WAYS TO FILL IT

One of the most common pieces of news a dentist gives you upon examination is that you have a cavity. In fact, 90 percent of American adults get cavities. In 2005 alone, 180 million cavities were filled. The good news is, though, today, cavities can be filled more quickly and painlessly than ever before.

Cavities are caused by plaque. Plaque causes decay and decay creates a hole in the tooth, which explains why they are called *cavities*. Whether the decay is new or buried under an old restoration, it needs to be removed, which, as you probably know, is done with a dentist's drill. The most common sites for decay occur in the contact area, in the deep grooves of the tooth or near the gum line or the root. If it's near the root, the dentist may first put in a liner of glass ionomer, composite resin, or other material to protect the nerve. If necessary, you may also be given an anesthetic.

The Restorative Options

Once the decay's been cleaned out of a cavity, the dentist evaluates how much of the tooth is left, and that determines what kind of restoration he'll put in there. The type of restoration used also depends on its location. For example, if it's in the aesthetic zone (the most visible front part of the smile), it needs to look natural and blend in. If it's in the back of the mouth, it needs to be strong and durable.

Direct Restoratives

Direct restoratives fit *directly* on the tooth (or teeth) once the decay is cleaned out. A filling is the smallest of the restorations, and a tooth can be filled with either silver amalgam or composite. Direct restoratives are also less costly than indirect restorations.

Composite

Composites are by far the most subtle restorations. Composites are made of a material, called bis-gma resin, which includes a type of glass filler particle in a resin base. A composite is sculpted either into a cavity or onto a tooth; it's then cured with a light and shaped in. The procedure is also known as bonding or a bonded restoration. When the decay is minor, a composite is an excellent choice.

The advantages of tooth-colored composites:
- Since it's contained within a tooth (as opposed to taking over an entire side or section of a tooth), it doesn't encounter much force.
- Its color blends in with your other teeth. But bear in mind that it's operator-sensitive; how good it looks depends on how good the dentist is who's placing it.
- It's kinder to the soft tissue than gold or silver amalgams.
- Unlike other fillings, composites actually chemically bond to your tooth structure, giving further support to your tooth.
- Less removal of the tooth's structure is required with composite fillings.

The downsides of composites:
- They don't last as long as the other options (five to ten years, usually), and can't withstand as much chewing force as the other options. However, as technology continues to improve, composites are getting better and stronger.

- Depending on their location, the composite materials can chip off.
- They can cost up to twice as much as silver amalgams. (Most dental insurance covers the cost of composites up to the price of the silver filling; then the patient must pay the difference.)

Silver

Silver amalgams consist of mercury mixed with silver, tin, zinc, and copper. It should be noted that silver amalgams are being used less and less because of the advancements in the arena of resin. With the many resin filling materials available, silver has become increasingly outdated.

The advantages of silver amalgam:
- It's nearly as durable as gold.
- It can withstand chewing forces.
- It's less expensive than gold, porcelain, and composite fillings.

The downsides of silver:
- Many patients don't like the look of silver in their mouths.
- Sometimes healthy parts of the tooth need to be removed to make room for the amalgam filling.
- Silver has the potential to crack and fracture more than other filling materials.
- A very small percentage of people (1 percent) are allergic to the mercury present in amalgam restora-

tions. The reaction is typically similar to a mild skin rash.

Indirect Restoratives

Indirect restoratives are made of either gold or porcelain. When an indirect restorative is required, an impression is first taken of the inside of the cavity-evacuated tooth. That impression is then sent to a lab, where a gold or porcelain piece (the restoration) is fabricated. Then it comes back to the dentist, who places it in the tooth; this usually requires two appointments.

Gold

Gold fillings are the Teflon of the filling family, but for all their power, they're equally garish. If the tooth is way in the back of the mouth, say, within a molar, where it will be well concealed, a gold filling will sustain the hard work it endures and its color won't offend.

The advantages of gold filling:

- When the tooth requires durability. Gold lasts at least ten and up to twenty-five years and doesn't corrode.

The downsides of gold:

- Gold is more expensive than other materials—the cost is up to ten times higher than that of an amalgam.
- Many patients don't like the look of gold in their mouths.
- Its placement requires at least two office visits.

- The ADA notes that if a gold filling is placed directly next to a silver amalgam, it can cause a sharp pain, called galvanic shock. While this is a rare occurrence, the interaction between the two metals and saliva can cause an electric current to occur.

Porcelain

Porcelains fall at the high end of all restorations. They're used in the aesthetic zone where gold is almost impermissible.

The advantages of porcelain:

- Porcelain as a material is very strong and sturdy; stronger than a composite.
- It's very kind to gum tissue.

The downsides of porcelain:

- Porcelain can only be used in a limited amount in a tooth. If the restoration is too big, a crown restoration has to be used instead.
- It's expensive.
- Although strong with up and down force, porcelain is weak under bending or shearing force and it can fracture under excessive loads.

THE SPECIALISTS

When you require treatment for something more than the common cavity, it usually requires that you see

MERCURY: A THING OF THE PAST OR AN OLD STANDBY?

Growing up, most of us who had cavities had them filled with amalgams made of silver, tin, mercury, and some other trace elements such as copper. While their aluminum-foil-like appearance wasn't the most attractive, they were durable (many last up to twenty years). Today, even though more attractive tooth-colored composite resins are available (and used by many dentists), the standard amalgam is what most practices still fill cavities with.

Theories of mercury leaking from cavities causing toxicity resulting in certain autoimmune diseases have spread far and wide in the dental world. But while high levels of mercury found in certain seafood have altered people's menu selections, its appearance in fillings is far less volatile. Although mercury by itself is classified as a toxic material, the mercury in an amalgam is chemically bound to other metals to make it stable and therefore safe for use in dental applications. In fact, amalgam is the most thoroughly studied and tested restorative material now used. The safety and effectiveness of amalgams have been reviewed by major U.S. and international scientific and health bodies, including the American Dental Association, the National Institutes of Health, the U.S. Public Health Service, the Centers for Disease Control and Prevention, the Food and Drug Administration, and the World Health Organization. All have concluded that mercury amalgam is a safe and effective material for restoring teeth.

a dental specialist. Ideally, your dentist can recommend good specialists, but if need be, call your local university's graduate dental school for references. Here's a rundown of the oral health specialists out there:

Prosthodontist

If you're contemplating restorative dentistry, changing old fillings, or sensitivities in the mouth, the super-restorative dentist is the prosthodontist, specially trained in the form and the function of teeth, and specifically in restoring them. A prosthodontist is a dentist who went for post-graduate training in these areas. (Note: A general dentist can also be an excellent restorative dentist with the proper training.)

Endodontist

An endodontist is specialty trained in diagnosing and treating problems associated with the inside of the tooth. If you need to have a root canal, it should be done by an endodontist.

Orthodontist

An orthodontist examines, diagnoses, and treats irregularities of tooth position and malrelations of jaws. If you or your child needs braces, you should seek an orthodontist.

Periodontist

If you have areas in your mouth that show symptoms of the supporting structure of the teeth—gum and bone—breaking down, your dentist will send you to a periodontist. This specialist examines, diagnoses, and treats the manifestations of gum problems. He'll eliminate the pockets (you will learn about these later), perform bone or tissue grafting, place implants, and meet any of the whole host of requirements necessary to heal any problems with the supporting structure of the teeth.

Oral Surgeon

The oral surgeon takes care of any surgical needs. Under this umbrella are biopsies and removing anything pathological in the mouth, including wisdom teeth. He's also trained to place implants, so you can choose between the oral surgeon and the periodontist for those.

THREE

THE RIGHT TOOLS TO MAINTAIN YOUR SMILE

THE EXPERT'S GUIDE TO THE BEST PRODUCTS FOR MAINTAINING YOUR SMILE

You splurge on the best moisturizer to help your skin stay younger longer, and you invest in a good pair of running shoes because you know that a not-so-good pair could mess up your ankles or feet. The products and tools you purchase for your smile should matter as much to you as the items you put on your face or wear on your body. Not only will they help you maintain a great smile—or even help you get a better one—but they won't cost even a fraction of what you spend on all that other stuff in your medicine cabinet or closet.

YOU *CAN* BUY BEAUTY, AND AT A REASONABLE PRICE

As the link between self-esteem and looking good continues to tighten, we continue to spend money on anything that promises to fix our imperfections. Anti-aging products are huge moneymakers, since we are a society obsessed with staying and looking young. But did you ever stop to think that a few small objects—a toothbrush, dental floss, and a tube of toothpaste—could do more for your looks than ten jars of La Mer?

The skin care department can get really confusing. AHA or anti-oxidant moisturizer? Micro-dermabrasion or acid peel? Eye cream or Botox? In the oral care world, it's far less confusing, and, nine times out of ten, far less expensive.

THE RIGHT TOOTHBRUSH

If dentists ruled the world, everyone would own an ultrasonic toothbrush. It gives you a professional clean feeling, right in your own bathroom. The plaque is brushed off the surface of the teeth with just the right amount of aggression, and the day's extrinsic stains get brushed off as well.

What's more, the latest models have a beeper installed that goes off every thirty seconds to signal when it's time to move on to the next quadrant in your mouth. The Sonicare Elite has two different settings, and Sonicare's latest, IntelliClean, has a built-in slot for a toothpaste "cartridge" to slip into, so the toothpaste is already inside the brush. Just a few pushes of a button send it directly into the brush. Ultrasonics can cost anywhere from $90 to $150. I've found that quality is often compromised in the lowest-priced brushes, but most of the ones in the middle price range are quite adequate.

Do You Actually Need a Rotating or Oscillating Toothbrush?

Thirty-one percent of Americans have one, but that doesn't necessarily mean you need one. It simply depends on how well you treat your teeth. So you probably already know the answer here. How well—and for how long—do you brush them? If you know that you're a lazy brusher—and denying it will only hurt you in the long run—then you need one. Time yourself next time you brush. If you clock in at less than a minute, you need one. According to a study done in 1998 by the *Journal of Clinical Dentistry,* most people do in fact need one since the average American's brushing time is thirty-nine seconds. As a professional, this number shocks me. You may be shocked, too . . . until you time yourself.

If you're still on the fence about whether you should use a rotating brush, ask your dentist and dental hygienist to grade you on your oral-care habits. They'll give you a straightforward and honest answer.

The Right Manual Brush

If you prefer to use a standard manual toothbrush, there are some characteristics you should look for when purchasing one.

- **Easy grip:** It should have a handle that's easy to grip and long enough so as not to make the action of brushing awkward.
- **Head space:** It should have a marginally small head so it can easily reach every spot.
- **Soft touch:** Its bristles should be soft with rounded ends and lie at a forty-five-degree angle to the teeth to allow you to easily and gently move it between the gum and teeth in a nonaggressive sideways motion.

BEWARE OF IMPORTS

Steer clear of the designer toothbrush. Those fancy toothbrushes sold at high-end pharmacies might look sexy and chic posing sinkside, but they're *not* friendly to your teeth. These European imports are made with bristles that are just too hard and abrading and could likely end up destroying your teeth's enamel. The future of manual toothbrushes lies with those that have replaceable heads. This innovation allows users to hold on to the higher-quality brushes by changing only the heads when necessary. Look for the GUM Protect Toothbrush and Fuchs EkoTec Toothbrushes. This is a strong trend, so keep an eye out for more makes, models, and improved designs.

SOFTENING UP

If your gum line is receding, if you have other gum sensitivity like oral ulcerations, or if you're undergoing chemotherapy, you should use an ultrasoft bristled toothbrush. The brand Biotène makes some especially soft brushes.

Manual brush recommendations: Colgate, Oral-B.

Electric brush recommendations: Sonicare Advance, Sonicare Elite, or Sonicare IntelliClean; Oral-B Professional Care.

The Toothbrush Owner's Manual

As a rule, it's a good idea to replace your toothbrush every thirty to forty-five days. (If the bristles begin to fray in less than forty-five days, ease up. You're brushing too aggressively!) That may seem wasteful, especially when you consider that most Americans replace theirs less than twice a year. But ponder this: Every time you brush, you're removing plaque from inside and between your teeth. That plaque is formed by bacteria, so the bacteria slide off your teeth and onto your toothbrush, where they nest.

The icing on this unappetizing cake is that about 30 to 40 percent of all toothbrushes actually harbor *E. coli* bacteria on them. *E. coli* bacteria can bring about gastrointestinal problems or infectious diseases. Still, so

---

TOOTHBRUSH SANITIZERS:
DENTAL DRY CLEANING

If the thought of bacteria on your toothbrush makes you squirm, there's an extra step you can take to ward against it. Toothbrush sanitizers are electronically powered sterilizing machines that steam-clean toothbrushes, and dry them with dry heat, virtually ridding them of any and all existing bacteria. Violight™ makes a hi-tech one that won many design awards. Brush sanitizers run anywhere from thirty to sixty dollars. Not only will they give you peace of mind, but they can extend the life of your toothbrush as well.

---

long as you rinse yours thoroughly and keep it in a spot where it can dry safely in open air, you really don't need to switch it more than every other month.

Other important points about your toothbrush are:

- Never share your toothbrush. It's like a bacteria swap meet.
- Change yours at both the start and at the end of any illness, even if it's something as innocuous as the common cold.
- Air-dry it nightly. This might seem obvious, but, believe it or not, some people toss theirs into the bottom of a dark drawer right after using it. A wet toothbrush in a dark enclosed area is just begging for more bacteria to hop on board and colonize.

- Always rinse your brush thoroughly (top and bottom, for at least ten seconds) to keep any suspicious creepy crawlies away. Toothpaste can leave behind a most unappetizing residue if you don't.

THE STRING SECTION

As with toothpastes, consumer options in dental floss are experiencing a boom. You can now find floss in several different textures—thick or thin, roped or ribbon-flat, waxed or nonwaxed. There are flosses that promise to whiten, strengthen tooth enamel, and reduce plaque. Flosses, like mini mouthwashes, also come flavored in everything from cinnamon to berry to even tea tree oil, deodorizing the area between teeth. In reality, though, none of these "specialty" flosses has enough actives to live up to its claims.

The best flosses are the PTFE types, which are fairly new to the market. *PTFE* stands for "polytetrafluoroethylene." Gore-Tex is a PTFE. Glide was the first of this kind to hit the market, and, in my opinion, it's the best floss you can get. The reason PTFE floss is so great is that it's made of a material similar to Teflon. It's like a tape, so it removes more plaque under the gum, and better than anyone else's. Plus, its flat shape allows it to easily snap through the contact (the spot where the two teeth touch each other from the side). This also means there's less chance of it shredding.

If you're all thumbs, a floss holder can help. It's a

Y-shaped little tool that holds the floss like a tiny suspension bridge, so you only need to direct it in, with a lot less need for finger coordination. You can buy the preloaded kind (for single use) or the kind you reload yourself each time you use it. There's a new brand, called Floss 'n Toss, which is a mini floss holder. It's shaped like a little C, and works basically the same way the larger floss holders do.

Especially reluctant flossers will be happy to learn that there are now even electric flossing devices. A piece of sturdy fishing-line-like nylon is vibrated between teeth in an oscillating motion. Waterpik makes one, Ultrasonex makes one, and Oral-B's new entry is called the Hummingbird.

The downside to an electric flosser is that it can be somewhat aggressive along the gum line. Overzealous flossing can actually change the shape of the gum tissue between your teeth, particularly in the aesthetic zone (the part of your smile that others see), and create dark triangles at the necks of teeth. If you elect to use an electric flossing device, look for the one that uses the fewest strokes per minute and always exercise care when using it.

EXTRA HELP

If your dental history consists of no more than a few cavities and the standard teenage orthodontics, regular brushing and flossing are usually a sufficient at-home regimen. But if you've had extensive work done, whether it was restorative dentistry, periodontal therapy, or implants (where teeth are literally attached to one another, offering no openings to slip floss up into), there is a subset group of specially designed devices to help reach between teeth at the gum line, making that critical area right where the tooth emerges easier to clean.

Proxy Brush

Proxy is a kind of slang name for brushes specifically designed to get between the necks of teeth. It's taken from the term *interproximal,* which means "between the necks of the teeth." This tiny, compact brush fits snugly between the necks horizontally. If your dentist ever put splinted crowns (crowns that are attached to one another) in your mouth, those splinted crowns are actually designed to allow this kind of brush to slip in between the gum line area below the contact. Proxy brushes are great at mechanically pushing bacteria and food out of the gum area to prevent future inflammation.

It's important to note that a proxy brush shouldn't be used on natural teeth because it could open a contact area and create a dark triangle. There's actually a name for this; it's called black triangle disease. Unless you've got splints (teeth splinted to one another), stick with floss.

Super Floss

Another great invention for splinted teeth is Super Floss, which is a rigid nylon that threads between the teeth at the gum line level, instead of slipping it down— or up—through the teeth. Threading the floss in this way prevents the risk of opening up what dentists refer to as "dark triangles" along the gum line.

Floss Threader

Floss threaders help slip the floss into tightly closed areas, such as beneath bridges or under orthodontic retainers.

Interdental Picks

The fancier version of a toothpick, these are made with either balsa wood or plastic to help mechanically remove plaque and food from between teeth. While it's great to want to get the plaque and food out of there, be sure to go easy on the area. Too much pushing and shoving could alter the shape of the line of the soft tissue, which could bring about black triangle disease mentioned earlier.

Rubber Tips

These are great for toning the soft tissue of the gums, especially the ones in the upper front that need to be massaged to stay tight and healthy. Rubber tips are also great tools for splinted teeth, since the rubber acts as a kind of squeegee, removing plaque and massaging the soft tissue. These should be used with the same amount of pressure that you'd give to a mascara wand—in other words, not very much.

Oral Irrigators

Oral irrigators have been around for years. They're at-home versions of those mini hoses your dentist uses to shoot water between your teeth. Most people know them by the top-selling brand, Waterpik. Oral irrigators really are quite effective in flushing out bacteria and food from between teeth and other hard-to-reach areas of the mouth, and water is certainly a rather harmless vehicle. In situations where you've got some inflammation, under the guidance of a professional, an oral irrigator's reservoir can be filled with an oral antiseptic liquid or an anti-bacterial to provide extra chemotherapeutic benefits to gums in need.

Recommendations: Waterpik products are old standbys. Hydro Floss also makes a solid product that adds a positive charge to the water and reverses its polarity, which helps prevent bacteria from sticking to root surfaces. Panasonic and Oral-B make smaller, more portable devices.

TOOTHPASTE OPTIONS

With so many toothpastes on the shelves, it is difficult to distinguish among them. This section will help you sort through the many choices and find what's right for you.

Ingredients

It takes dozens of ingredients to help toothpaste look, taste, feel, and perform the way it's supposed to. Take a few moments to educate yourself about ingredients in toothpastes that can help or hinder your oral health.

Fluoride: Everyone should use toothpaste that contains fluoride. Fluoride helps prevent decay and improves gum health. It also decreases bacteria's ability to stick to root surfaces. And fluoride improves a tooth's overall hardness, fortifying it, both topically on the tooth and internally. During the time that children's adult teeth are growing in, fluoride plays a big part in their formation. Fluoride turns a hydroxyapatite molecule (a basic building block of enamel) into a fluorapatite one, which makes the tooth much more resistant to breakdown from decay. Fluoride has been proven to decrease decay by 60 percent. Of course, as with all actives and drugs, the exact dosage is critical for effectiveness and safety. Ask your dentist what your ideal levels of fluoride are. Too much of it can cause fluorosis in teeth, resulting in pitting and even brown stains.

Triclosan: This anti-bacterial is used in everything from detergents to deodorants to, yes, toothpaste. Like sodium lauryl sulfate (and often fluoride), triclosan is on the ecofriendly zealots' "hit list."

Questions have arisen about how smart it is to use this

THE SODIUM LAURYL SULFATE DEBATE

Foaming agents help remove plaque and deodorize the mouth. They also keep toothpaste thick so that it doesn't pour out of the mouth. The most commonly used foaming agent is sodium lauryl sulfate (SLS). SLS has some controversy around it because its usage has been linked to everything from cataracts to liver and kidney damage to certain types of cancer. But since investigations by respectable publications (including the *Washington Post* and the *Berkeley Wellness Newsletter*) have come up with no evidence linking the foaming agent to any of those maladies, and because there is such a small amount of it in toothpastes, I believe it is virtually harmless.

Studies have shown, however, that SLS can play a role in increased incidence of canker sores. If you find you're prone to them, or any kind of oral sensitivity, you should choose a toothpaste that does not contain this ingredient.

anti-microbial every day, since certain triclosan-resistant bacteria have been discovered. Much the way we avoid taking antibiotics too frequently because our resistance to them would weaken, if triclosan is used too much, it can remove the powers of certain friendly bacteria in the mouth. Products from lines such as Tom's of Maine, GoSMILE, and Kiss My Face replace triclosan with natural alternatives in their oral care products.

Gantrez: Gantrez is an ingredient that allows triclosan to remain on teeth for a longer period of time, thereby protecting them for several hours throughout the day. Colgate Total contains gantrez.

Sweeteners: Sweeteners improve the taste of the toothpaste. Saccharine is a commonly used one. There are also the sugar alcohols, sorbitol and xylitol, which are actually neither sugar nor alcohol. Go figure. Xylitol not only prevents toothpaste from tasting bad, but also helps prevent cavity formation, so many dentists give it a gold star.

Whitening Toothpastes

Whitening is the number one reason people buy toothpaste today, so it should come as no surprise that the top-selling toothpastes are all of the whitening variety (whitening toothpastes are now a five-hundred-million-dollar-a-year industry), knocking cavity prevention off its long-standing top slot. Usually containing buffers to help wipe away extrinsic stains, they may also contain a form of hydrogen peroxide. Calprox (calcium peroxide) is a popular one, as is carbamide peroxide. But do they really whiten?

Since neither the FDA nor the ADA actually defines what *whitening* means, nor do they regulate the claims stamped on the sides of toothpaste boxes, companies can include the term *whitening* with no regard for whether their products actually do whiten. In fact, most whitening toothpastes don't really whiten. In order for a toothpaste to truly whiten teeth, it has to contain a high concentration (at least 6 percent) of the active ingredient hydrogen peroxide. And currently, none does.

Furthermore, the active ingredient needs to remain on teeth for twenty to thirty minutes in order for it to actually do something. You would need to brush for at least ten to fifeen minutes a day with the average whitening toothpaste for at least fifteen to twenty days in a row in order to see any whitening improvements. What whitening toothpastes can do is gently polish off stains with buffers, such as silica or bicarbonate, and prevent stains from clinging to teeth with ingredients like fluoride or pyrophosphates.

Breath-Freshening Toothpastes

While just about every toothpaste contains ingredients to freshen breath, some target halitosis more seriously. Real, honest-to-goodness breath freshening can happen only when the bacteria that cause bad breath can actually be locked down. If bad breath is a big problem and you feel compelled to use an anti-bacterial toothpaste, limit its use to once or twice a week. Actives such as chlorine dioxide (in Oxyfresh and Biotène toothpastes) do help keep the bacterial numbers under control. For the rest of the week, supplement with a deodorizing toothpaste, such as Arm & Hammer baking soda toothpaste. It contains natural deodorizing ingredients like sodium bicarbonate or calcium bicarbonate.

THE ABRASION INDEX

Toothpastes are measured by their relative dentin abrasivity, or RDA (not to be confused with the other RDA, recommended daily allowance). Check out how yours stacks up against the rest. The thing to notice here is that, just as you don't want a toothbrush with bristles that are too coarse, you don't want your toothpaste to be highly abrasive. Most professionals recommend using one with a low RDA rating, especially if your teeth are sensitive.

RDA Rating of Most Toothpastes
Close-Up: 218
Aim: 185
Aquafresh Whitening: 113
Colgate Platinum: 106
Crest: 106
Mentadent: 103
Tom's of Maine: 93
Colgate: 68
CloSYS II: 53
Enamel Saver: 44
GoSMILE AM/PM: 110

Gingivitis- and Plaque-Removing Toothpastes

When your gums become inflamed, you need to bring them back to their normal condition. Once plaque reaches into the gum and gets underneath, it can lead to gum inflammation and, over time, bone loss (chronic bone loss is periodontal disease), then finally tooth loss. First, have your dental professional evaluate you. Chances are, he will recommend a gingivitis-fighting toothpaste. Most of them, including Colgate Total, contain specific anti-bacterial ingredients such as triclosan.

Should you prefer to take the more natural route, both tea tree oil and zinc help increase the ability to rid the area of plaque-related bacteria. One such option is Desert Essence Natural Tea Tree Oil Toothpaste (which does not contain triclosan). There are also prescription-only toothpastes available through your dentist.

Whatever special paste you choose, be sure that once the soft tissue (gum) has returned to its healthy state, you switch back to a toothpaste that doesn't contain an active gingival-fighting ingredient. A less stringent toothpaste will maintain a better balance in your mouth, which, in turn, will strengthen your immune response and your mouth's ability to fight infection.

Tartar-Control Toothpastes

Tartar-control toothpastes contain sodium pyrophosphates, which help prevent more tartar from forming. But the real problem of gum inflammation and periodontal disease is caused by bacteria forming under the gum. At the end of the day, we're talking about fighting bacteria and preventing gums from becoming inflamed. But since these toothpastes deal more with the accu-

HOW IMPORTANT IS THE ADA SEAL?

Since 1934, the American Dental Association has been awarding its Seal of Acceptance to dental products that are safe and effective. The seal is valid for three years, and then a company has to reapply to continue wearing it. If the product is altered in any way, the company must resubmit it for review and approval. When a product is submitted for the seal, its company hands over data on clinical and laboratory studies to support its claims on safety and efficacy, its ingredient list, plus any advertising and promotional materials. Then a consortium of more than one hundred consultants and staff scientists review the product's effectiveness to determine whether it meets ADA standards.

At present, close to five hundred consumer dental products carry the ADA seal, including toothpaste, dental floss, mouth rinses, and toothbrushes. Whether this seal is really necessary is debatable. Some cynics see no reason for it, in this age of advanced technology, except as a marketing ploy. But many consumers still feel safer when they buy an oral care product bearing the ADA seal.

mulated tartar on the enamel than with that on and under the gum, only a dentist and a dentist's tools can remove the unwanted stuff that's already made itself at home.

Desensitizing Toothpastes

Sixty percent of the American population have sensitivity issues with their teeth. When the tooth's nerve is exposed, it becomes sensitive to different conditions, such as sweetness and temperature. This recession can occur from either environmental factors or heredity. The recession prompts those tiny dentinal tubules to transmit an impulse to the nerve. Desensitizing toothpastes contain active ingredients such as potassium nitrate that seal up the tubules, preventing fluid from flowing there, which is what sets off the sensitivity. Potassium nitrate is a most effective desensitizing agent when receding gums expose root. In order for a toothpaste to be effective, however, it must contain a concentration of about 5 percent potassium nitrate or any of the other active ingredients. An example is Sensodyne.

Children's Toothpastes

If you've got kids, you know how important it is to emphasize proper brushing habits. There are some great-tasting children's toothpastes that not only use flavoring, but also have anti-cariogenic (translation: decay-preventing) effects. Look for ingredient names such as xylitol and sorbitol. Products containing these may be a bit more expensive, but just think of all the money you could be saving in cavity-filling costs down the road! Try Tom's of Maine Natural Anticavity Fluoride Toothpaste in Outrageous Orange-Mango and Silly Strawberry.

BAD BREATH FIGHTERS

Having a breath freshener in one's toothpaste isn't enough for most people to combat bad breath. As oral care progresses, so do the options to help fight bad breath and keep its causes at bay.

Tongue Scrapers

The tongue is your breath's worst enemy. Even more than those crevices between your teeth, your tongue stores within its fibers loads of bacteria that cause bad breath.

It wasn't long ago that tongue brushing and tongue scraping were pretty much unheard of; now most hygienists tell all patients to brush or scrape their tongues. The most lethal area of the tongue is, unfortunately, toward the back, where most of the bacteria are harbored. While thorough tongue brushing is great at removing the bacteria, it can induce the gag reflex. That's when a tongue scraper comes in handy. Some resemble spoons; others look more like small windshield wipers, but the best-designed tongue scrapers are flexible enough to maneuver easily and have ragged edges to help grab the VSCs (volatile sulfur compounds produced by bacteria hiding within the recesses of the tongue) from within the tongue. Your dental professional should have—or at the very least be familiar with—the various tongue scrapers, and can show you how to use them effectively.

Mouthwashes

Another way to fight bad breath is to use mouthwash. This cooling liquid washes over you and your VSCs like a little ocean wave of mint. But there's a mental trick that the big names of the mouthwash industry play on you: You believe that if your mouth feels cool, then your breath is fresh. And it actually is—for ten minutes, maybe. Most mouthwashes only perform for a brief period. The standard mouthwash comes and goes just about as quickly as that ocean wave.

Most mouthwashes contain these components:

- An active bacterium-fighting ingredient such as zinc gluconate, quaternary ammonium compounds, or cetylpyridinium chloride, which is found in Cepacol and GoSMILE Daily.
- A flavoring agent such as saccharine or glycerine.
- Astringents, like zinc chloride, to provide a pleasant-tasting sensation and shrink tissues.
- Ethyl alcohol, ranging from 18 to 27 percent.
- Water.
- Phenolic compounds (found in Listerine).

Listerine and Scope contain high levels of alcohol in their formulas—in fact, they surpass both red and white wine. Believe it or not, alcohol is often used to make the product more appealing; if these rinses contained no alcohol, they would have a murky look to them. But alcohol does so many bad things to a mouth.

PHENOLS: THE OTHER ALCOHOL

Some mouthwashes (including Listerine) contain phenols—types of alcohol that have widely been considered toxic because they're susceptible to being absorbed by lungs and skin, potentially resulting in caustic burns as well as kidney and liver damage and hyperactivity. When choosing a mouthwash, avoid anything containing this ingredient.

High levels (27 percent in Listerine) dry out the mouth's soft tissue and can cause burning sensations in teeth, gums, and cheeks—a condition called mucosal irritation. Also, the higher the level of alcohol in a rinse, the more sloughing occurs. More sloughing brings about more food for bacteria, which increases bacterial levels, which increases the sulfur levels of bad breath. It also destroys any resin technology that's been performed on the teeth, such as bonding or veneers.

A good alternative is natural mouthwashes, which are typically alcohol- and sugar-free. Many of the natural ones use baking soda as a natural abrasive to remove stains, plus pure mint oils or other essential oils, or even ginger for flavoring. Look for alcohol-free mouthwashes, such as Tom's of Maine, Crest Pro-Health, and a soon-to-be-released alcohol-free product from Scope.

Anti-Bacterial, Oxygenating Rinses

Oxygen inhibits bacterial growth. Ingredients that oxygenate include chlorine dioxide and natural zinc compounds, such as zinc gluconate and zinc chloride.

Three reputable oxygenating mouthwashes are TheraBreath PLUS Oral Rinse, BreathRx, and Oxyfresh Power Rinse.

These rinses are so powerful on bacteria that I suggest only using them a few times a week, supplementing the other days with the more standard bacterium-fighting rinses.

Therapeutic Rinses

Therapeutic rinses contain specific active ingredients that target specific oral problems. Usually, they're prescription-level products, and so should be used only as prescribed by your dentist, and only as long as the dentist recommends.

Therapeutic rinses address both short-term and long-term needs.

Short-term needs:
- **Post-perio:** After periodontal surgery, your periodontist might prescribe a rinse such as Peridex to keep bacteria away. Peridex stains teeth, though, so be sure to make up for that with an at-home gentle whitening product.

- **Gingivitis or plaque:** Anti-plaque rinses use a variety of ingredients to loosen and detach plaque from tooth surfaces above the gum line.

  These usually contain the active ingredient chlorhexidine, known to be the most effective plaque-fighting drug. Chlorhexidine inhibits the formation of plaque and calculus. This kind of rinse should be used only for a short time because it can seriously stain teeth. So even during this brief period, you should use a type of at-home whitening product to control the staining.

- **Dry mouth** (which could also be long term, in some cases): People with severe dry mouth (medically called xerostomia) usually acquire this condition from having gone through radiation therapy. Oral rinses, such as Biotène, contain natural enzymes to rebalance the bacteria in the mouth, encouraging a moister environment.

Long-term needs:

- **Cavities:** Anti-cavity rinses with fluoride usually contain 0.05 percent sodium fluoride or 0.1 percent stannous fluoride and have been clinically proven to fight up to 50 percent more of the bacteria that cause cavities. Many dentists, though, consider the use of fluoride toothpaste alone to be more than adequate protection against cavities.

- **Smokers:** Smoker's mouthwashes dissolve and remove stubborn tobacco tar stains from teeth. They use glycerine (oil) and salt-based ingredients (sodium lauryl sulfate and sodium benzoate) in an alcohol- and water-based solution.

- **Dry mouth:** Dry mouth also happens to people who have Sjögren's syndrome, a condition in which immune cells attack and destroy the glands that produce tears and saliva. There are tablets called Salagen, which stimulate the salivary glands.

GO EASY ON THE SAUCE

Many prescribed rinses' higher levels of active ingredients can cause a number of side effects, including aphthous ulcers (canker sores), sodium retention, root sensitivity, soreness, numbness, changes in taste sensation, painful mucosal erosions, and staining.

Mouth Sprays

It all began with the Binaca blast. Like a portable mouthwash, one shot of a breath spray is quick and easy—it can be done anytime, anywhere, giving your mouth that immediate burst of cool. But most breath sprays are also no more than quick-fix bacterial camouflages. Sprays containing the true actives are just starting to hit the market. Look for the ingredients that I've already mentioned—the zinc compounds and CPC (cetylpyridinium chloride) or chlorine dioxide—on the labels of this new group.

Most breath sprays contain alcohol and saccharine,

> ## HOME COOKING
>
> If you can do without the minty flavoring, you can make
> your own basic mouth rinse by mixing a saline solution
> (either half a teaspoon of salt and eight ounces of water,
> or, for a strong solution, half a teaspoon of salt in four
> ounces water) or a sodium bicarbonate one (half a
> teaspoon of baking soda and eight ounces of water).

which are the worst ingredients you can put in your
mouth. Saccharine is a sugar substitute, and you probably already are aware that it's been at the forefront of
a cancer controversy for two decades.

The fact that breath sprays containing both alcohol
and a potentially harmful sugar substitute *still* exist is
something I find hard to believe. We are long overdue
for a change in this department. In the meantime,
there are a couple of sprays on the market that I recommend to patients: BreathRx and TheraBreath Power
Drops.

Breath Mints

The majority of breath mints usually only make the
problem worse. Why? Because 95 percent of breath
mints are packed with sugar or sugar alcohols, which
feed the bacteria that cause decay. These sugar alcohols
aren't really bad for you (xylitol even helps prevent

decay), but they certainly don't deliver that promised fresh breath. A natural alternative is Ricola Herb Drops.

Chewing Gum

The great thing about chewing gum is that it initiates salivary flow. Saliva is filled with fantastic natural protective enzymes and compounds that prevent decay and gum disease by flushing the mouth and dislodging the various bacteria in there. Still, most gum is laced with sugar, which, as you know, causes decay.

If you must chew, chew sugarless. But the next time you pop a piece of chewing gum in your mouth, consider the wear and tear it's putting on your jaw system. While we're told that chewing gum removes foods from the mouth and the surfaces of the teeth, that positive act is far outweighed by the abuse it's doing to your jaw. Teeth usually only come together for seven to ten minutes a day under normal functions (when we chew our food). But daily gum chewing puts them together for literally hours each day, and chewing and overuse of the teeth and jaw muscles can eventually lead to temporomandibular joint (TMJ) disorder and myofascial pain dysfunction (MPD).

There are two things that cause the destruction of the mouth: plaque and force. Though you might not have considered it before, chewing gum is a forceful action. Whistle instead. Or, better yet, smile.

FOUR

GETTING TO KNOW YOUR MOUTH

arlier you learned that it takes significantly fewer muscles to smile than it does to frown—about seventeen versus forty-three. The mouth alone has eight different muscles, ranging from those responsible for moving the lips to the ones that raise and lower the jaw. Among the smile muscles, on the other side of the lips, the tongue lashes around against thirty or so teeth and a reservoir of saliva keeps everything lubricated, including the soft tissue that holds the structure together.

The mouth is the most highly functioning body part. All of its uses—eating, kissing, speaking, breathing, and, of course, smiling—are key to human functioning. Still, most of us take it for granted. We expect our teeth to chop our food for us when we're hungry; we rely on our tongue to flap away when we communicate. And we certainly count on our smile to get us what we want, whether it's a friendly returned greeting, a job, or overall acceptance in everyday life. But how well do you know the mouth's parts? How familiar are you with its characteristics and quirks?

Teeth are so much more than pretty, shiny chips. They may be no bigger than small pearls, but each one is a rather impressive and elaborate little structure. Their complexity is what makes them such formidable equipment.

A tooth is divided into three parts:

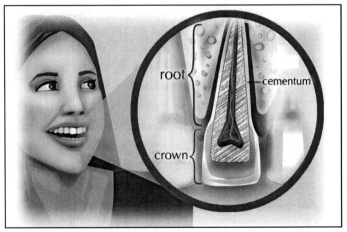

fig. 4.1

- **The root,** which is the foundation of the tooth. It's hidden below the gum line.
- **The cementum,** which is the layer of bone-like tissue that covers the outer surface of the root.
- **The crown,** which is the majority of the tooth and the part that's visible.

The body of the tooth consists of three layers: the enamel, the dentin, and the pulp.

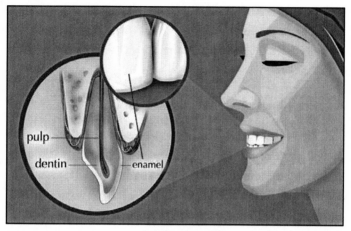

fig. 4.2

ENAMEL: TOOTH INSULATOR

The enamel is a thin layer of calcified material that covers the crown's surface, and it's responsible for that translucent glow that teeth have. Enamel is composed of enamel rods that look like, well, rods, but they're very tiny and there are hundreds of them threaded in there. Each rod is composed of a mineral called hydroxyapatite; this, in turn, is made up of a matrix of calcium and phosphate crystals. The tighter the matrix's structure, the harder the enamel is. And you want your enamel to be hard. The thing about enamel is that, no matter how "loose" its structure, it is always going to be the hardest substance in your entire body.

Enamel's Worst Enemy

Since it's almost 100 percent mineral, anything that can de-mineralize enamel is bad. That means acids, such as lemons or orange juice, or a diet that's high in proteins, which basically ignite acids already existing in the mouth.

DENTIN: COLOR AND OPACITY PROVIDER

The dentin lies just beneath the enamel and is the largest part of the tooth. This bone-like substance is comprised of minerals, water and protein. (While enamel is almost all mineral, dentin is about half mineral, half organic.) What's more important to know is that your tooth's color comes from the dentin. The condition of your dentin determines how bright—or not—that color will appear.

Dentin's Weakness

Overuse of at-home whitening products can be dentin's downfall. Oversaturation of peroxide on teeth can vaporize the particles within the dentin, called chromophores, that make up a tooth's opacity and color.

PULP: NUTRITION SUPPLIER, SENSATION MESSENGER

At the heart of the tooth is the pulp, which is first and foremost the blood supplier to the tooth. Blood travels from the pulp down to the dentin along mini pipelines called odontoblastic tubules, delivering nourishment. Along with feeding the dentin, it's also the pulp's job to transmit nerve impulses to the dentin.

Pulp's Weakness

As soon as bacteria get into the sterile pulp, it dies. The necrotic debris of the dying vital pulp tissue causes the body to think that a foreign substance has invaded, which sets off an immune response. More on that later.

THE BIGGER PICTURE: HOW IT'S ALL CONNECTED

Teeth may have their own structure, but they aren't just attached to the gums by some kind of bodily glue or something—unless, of course, they're dentures.

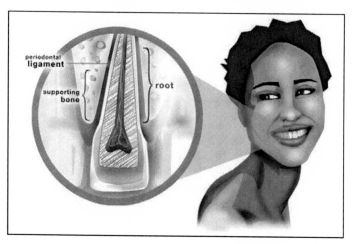

fig. 4.3

Rather, a tooth is attached to a bone. You can't see this bone—it's hidden under the gum. Above the bone, the gum is bound down to the root as well as the bone through a network of interlacing fibers, called periodontal ligaments. Periodontal ligaments are also what connect a tooth to the bone. The ligaments extend under the entire gum tissue, spreading over the whole of the bone as well as the roots of the teeth. Going even deeper, within the ligaments are thousands of tiny fibers that stretch from the bone to the root surface of the tooth, so they not only keep the tooth attached to everything but also cushion the teeth and act as a kind of shock absorber for them. Imagine if your teeth had no "give." Things would be pretty stiff and fragile in your mouth if this fiber network didn't exist.

INSIDER INFO

The flexibility of the periodontal ligaments is what makes the science of orthodontia possible. These ligaments provide teeth with the ability to shift their position somewhat and get realigned better.

In-Between Spaces

Between each tooth is a little space that extends ever so slightly up within the gum line between the tooth and the bone. It's called a gingival sulcus. This little space size should measure somewhere between one and three millimeters deep. Sometimes, usually due to poor oral hygiene, a sulcus can become larger or deeper, like five or six millimeters deep and greater. When that happens, it then becomes what's called a pocket. You never want your sulcuses to become pockets. (Gum health will be covered in more detail later in the book.)

Teeth are mapped out in a number system that's been used throughout all of modern times. Surely you've overheard your dentist and dental hygienist conferring about some decay they see on number 15, or noting that they need to do an X-ray on number 10. Most adults have between twenty-eight and thirty-two teeth, depending on whether or not their wisdom teeth have been removed.

While they may not exactly mirror each other, each tooth ideally has a mate across from it on the opposing jaw. The upper jaw is called the maxilla and the lower jaw, the mandible.

Wisdom Teeth

The farthermost back teeth are the wisdom teeth (also called the third molars). They're shaped like a crown with four cusps and were specifically designed that way to mash food. Thanks to evolution, we don't need them anymore. Yet we still get them, and they often grow in with annoying complications. They're either impacted, or they grow in sideways or only partially. It's practically a rite of passage to get them removed, usually somewhere between the late teens and the early twenties. But people get them removed at all ages. Ultimately, if they don't cause you discomfort, your wisdom teeth can remain. If and when they do bother you, though, they should be taken out. Your dental professional is the one to make this call.

The Mashing Molars

The first and second molars are the largest teeth in the mouth. They're mostly used for mashing food into small pieces, which helps our digestive system run more smoothly. But because they're so far back and more difficult to reach cleaning-wise, they're the likeliest to develop decay and those gingival pockets. Therefore, they're also the teeth that most commonly require root canals, crowns, and bridges. Still, without your molars, your face would basically collapse. The posterior molars support the front teeth vertically. Losing them would place all the pressure on your front teeth, and over time, the lower jaw would just close in, leaving the lower part of your face with no support. If this isn't a good enough reason to pay special attention to them, I don't know what is.

The Versatile Premolars

Next to the molars are the eight premolars, two on each side, top and bottom. These are also called the bicuspids, and they, along with the canines, rip food apart as well as help with the mashing. When you see someone smile in profile, the premolars are the ones that stand out from that angle. They're both the earliest to show signs of decay as well as the teeth most likely to suffer from aggressive brushing and gum recession. So treat them well, but be gentle.

The Superstrong Canines

Also called the cuspids and the eyeteeth, the canines are next to the premolars. Each of the quadrants has one canine. Though they may be smaller than animal canines, they are nevertheless the strongest and most stable of all of our teeth. Canines are critical because they help separate the back teeth from excessive amounts of force when you're chewing. They're often referred to as the transition teeth since they create the bifurcation between the front teeth and the back teeth. Their positioning is also critical in making sure that a bite works smoothly and efficiently (in dental verbiage, your bite is called your occlusion). Despite their power and strength, canines commonly suffer from gum recession because of their prominence in the dental arch.

The Dominating Incisors

There are two kinds of incisors, lateral and central. The lateral incisors live next to the canines, one per quadrant. The centrals are the two flattest and widest teeth, and they dominate (or should ideally dominate) the smile, front and center. (There are also two central incisors on the bottom but, unlike the upper centrals, the lower ones are just part of the lower lineup and aren't nearly as visible.) While their sharp edges are good for cutting, they are vulnerable, and the most likely to be injured. Great centrals are what make a great smile a *great smile*. If you've got a pair of big, healthy centrals, you've most likely already got a great smile.

THE SUM OF THE PARTS

So, as you now see, every tooth plays its part. Every tooth is important. Keep that in mind the next time you brush and floss. Think about which ones tend to be overbrushed; think about which ones get neglected. And just watch how your brushing and flossing routine changes.

FIVE

THE BASICS
REVIEWED

DON'T TAKE THAT SMILE FOR GRANTED

No matter how much time and money you invest in dental work, if you don't take care of your teeth and mouth on your own, your oral structures will gradually weaken, then fall apart. It might not seem possible for that to happen today, but improper flossing and brushing will catch up with you eventually.

I've got a question for you: How well do you think you clean your teeth? If you answer these five questions as honestly as you can, you'll be able to see how well—or how poorly—you stack up on the dental hygiene scale.

1. How many times a day do you brush your teeth?

    a. Once in the morning; sometimes at night.

    b. It's the first thing I do when I wake up, and last thing I do before bed.

    c. In the morning, at bedtime, and often after lunch.

    d. My toothbrush is my lifeline. I brush my teeth as often as I go to the bathroom.

2. How long do you spend brushing your teeth?

    a. About twenty seconds, but I do a great job. My mouth feels very clean afterward.

    b. Nearly a minute. I heartily brush both the uppers, then the lowers.

    c. I time myself or I consciously do some pre-bedtime chore while I brush, like turning out all the lights in the house or watching the weather report on the local news.

    d. I usually brush for about five minutes.

3. How attentive are you when you're brushing?

    a. Not very.

    b. I'm smiling into that mirror the entire time I brush. That's how I learned when I was a kid, and I've fared pretty well by it.

    c. I angle my brush to get into the crevices and massage the gums.

    d. My teeth never cease to fascinate me. Sometimes I stop and just inspect and inspect after brushing each tooth. So what if that means one less hour of sleep?

4. How aggressive are you when you brush?

   a. Very! If I'm going to brush them, they're in for a serious scrubbing!

   b. My wrists and fingers are in excellent shape thanks to the strength I put into my brushing technique.

   c. They may be sturdy teeth, but they need to be treated gently. What's more important is reaching into those hard-to-get spots and giving them adequate cleaning.

   d. Doesn't the brush do all the work?

5. Flossing is . . .

   a. Something I do the day before I'm seeing my dental hygienist. It's painful and often causes my gums to bleed.

   b. Something I do when I remember. I do it about as often as I vacuum.

   c. A part of my daily teeth-cleaning routine. I floss once a day, usually at night before bed.

   d. I carry floss with me and use it after every meal, especially when there's steak or corn on the cob involved.

TALLYING YOUR SCORE

For every A answer, give yourself 5 points.
For every B answer, give yourself 4 points.
For every C answer, give yourself 3 points.
And for every D answer, give yourself 1 point.

Points Chart: How Do You Stack Up?
5–8: Squeaky clean.
8–15: Room for improvement.
15–20: Pay more attention.
20–25: Get serious now!

Many people—particularly women—devote a lot of time and money to their faces, but too often neglect their teeth and gums. You should be paying just as much attention to your smile as you do to your skin! At the same time, it's important not to go overboard. Conscientious care is one thing, but obsessive tending to your teeth is another. No matter what your score, though, a quick review of the basics when it comes to oral care is always beneficial.

PLAQUE ATTACK

Plaque is a smile's number one enemy. If plaque isn't diligently brushed or flossed away, it can cause everything from enamel breakdown to gingivitis and periodontal disease.

Plaque is a sticky film of bacteria that covers teeth. After you eat, the bacteria release acids that attack tooth enamel. And if you eat sugary foods without cleaning well afterward, plaque thrives on that sugar. The more sugar you eat, the greater the amount of acid is produced in your mouth. As soon as it accumulates, acids will start to break the enamel down, de-mineralizing its protective coating and encouraging cavities to form.

When plaque stays on teeth, it begins to harden. Long-term plaque eventually turns into calculus or, as it's more commonly known, tartar. At this point, brushing and cleaning between teeth becomes more difficult because tartar accumulates and hardens above the gum line. The more your dental hygienist scrapes away on your teeth at the edges of your gums, the more plaque has stiffened into stubborn tartar.

Once plaque attacks the gums, gingivitis sets in and inflames them, causing them to redden, swell, and bleed. Since plaque doesn't stay still, it can creep below the gum line, and once it's there, it causes the gums to separate from the teeth. This sets the stage for eventual bone and tooth loss.

The thing is, there's really no need to ever have to experience cavities, de-mineralization, gingivitis, or bone loss. Plaque is easy to control—you just need to know how.

Maybe you're not doing it right.

BRUSHING 101

Sure, you brush your teeth twice a day. You may even brush for the required two minutes. But has anyone ever taught you exactly how to brush?

In chapter 3, I offered guidance on choosing the right toothbrush. Now it's time to concentrate on technique, which actually matters much more than having the right brush.

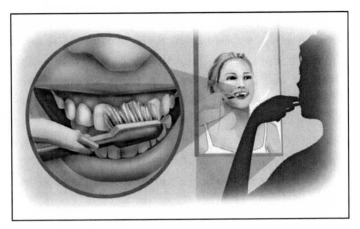

fig. 5.1

- **It's all in the wrist:** To begin, hold the toothbrush at a forty-five-degree angle to the tooth, so that the bristles gently move between the spaces and between the gum and the tooth in a gentle sideways motion. Next, sweep the brush up, then down. This movement will move the bacteria away from the critical area around the gum.

A LITTLE GOES A LONG WAY

Although toothpaste commercials show actors squirting huge swirls of toothpaste onto their toothbrushes, you really don't need more than a pea-size amount to do the job. More than that, and you're just wasting it. Kids need even less—about the size of the tip of a match, in fact.

- **Cover all bases:** It's imperative that you work on all surfaces, including the cheek surface by the upper teeth, the inner surface on the upper teeth, and the same for the bottom ones.
- **Chill out:** Don't take your frustrations out on your teeth. If you find your gums reddening after you brush, you're brushing too hard.
- **Time factor:** Brushing should take at least two minutes—that's critical to keep everything in there healthy and plaque-free. Count it out or set a timer— just don't stop before the two-minute mark.
- **Three times a brusher:** Ideally, you should brush your teeth when you wake up, at bedtime, and after every meal. But three times a day is a pretty good average to keep.

BABY BRUSHING

Healthy first teeth also contribute to proper alignment of the jawbones and eventual bite. As soon as that first baby tooth appears, a child's teeth (or tooth) must be brushed twice a day. In the beginning, you can wrap a piece of gauze around your finger and rub it across the teeth; no toothpaste is necessary until around the time of a child's third birthday. Before using a toothpaste that contains fluoride, check with your dentist. If your child is already getting fluoride supplements or drinks a lot of fluoridated water, don't use fluoridated toothpaste. If your dentist recommends fluoride toothpaste, only use a match-tip-size dab. Kids like to swallow toothpaste.

FLOSSING PROMOTES
TOOTH LONGEVITY

If you don't floss your teeth on a daily basis, you might as well start saving up for dentures. I cannot emphasize its importance enough. We all know we're supposed to do it, yet about 90 percent of us don't floss daily.

What your brushing can't reach, flossing can. It removes food particles and plaque that elude your toothbrush since the little stuff often hides behind and between the teeth. In fact, dentists consider it even more crucial in the prevention of tooth decay and periodontal disease than brushing. But, just like brushing incorrectly, flossing incorrectly can do more harm than good. Make sure you're doing it right.

Flossing Correctly

- Rip off about eighteen inches of the floss and wrap it around your pointer or middle finger. Wind the remaining floss around the same finger of the opposite hand, so you've got about seven inches between each hand.

- Pick a spot to start and make that your designated starting place, so you'll get into the routine of it. Most people pick the space between their two centrals or the molar farthest in the back. I suggest you start on the upper right and work around the mouth to the lower right.

- Direct the floss up between your teeth, and once it's in place, hold it taut. Use a sawing motion as you glide it between your teeth.

- Next, you need to get the floss under the soft tissue, so move it under there in a C-shaped fashion, gliding it back and forth. This will remove the plaque from those critical spaces between the teeth without doing any damage to that sometimes sensitive soft tissue. If you hold it instead in a vertical U position and pull it up into the soft tissue, you can actually do damage.

- Should your floss get stuck, don't tug on it to get it out. Just slide it out toward you from between the teeth, then reposition it and try again. Repeat the same process with each of your teeth.

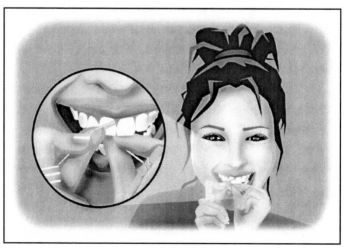

fig. 5.2

No Excuses

If the idea of flossing just bores you and you'd rather skip it, I bet I can change your attitude. Run the floss through a few nooks between your teeth. Now smell it. Nice, huh? That unappetizing bacterial smell is what you're subjecting those around you to if you don't floss. So you're not only hurting your teeth, but hurting others around you as well. And all the Altoids in the world won't mask it!

FLOSS FOR YOUR LIFE

There is a direct link between flossing and the prevention of heart disease. Countless studies have proven that poor dental cleaning and a lack of flossing can lead to heart disease. Researchers recently found that diseased gums released higher levels of bacterial pro-inflammatory components into the bloodstream. These components can find their way to other organs, including the heart, and increase their risk of failure.

There is clear evidence that periodontal disease is implicated in promoting the formation of lesions in blood vessel walls. This translates into an increased risk for major cardiovascular and cerebrovascular (stroke) events.

GET YOUR BREATH UNDER CONTROL

A study published in *Chain Drug Review* in October 2003 revealed that most Americans are obsessed with having bad breath. At least 90 percent of people between sixteen and forty feel that having bad breath is "the worst social mistake one can make." That's big.

These same people also say they constantly chew gum and mints to freshen their breath. But ironically, unless they're sugarless, gum and mints actually promote bad breath. Don't lose hope, though. There are ways to adequately attack bad breath.

When Breath Goes Bad

Nine times out of ten, bad breath is related to the condition of your mouth's interior, specifically the type of bacteria that reside—and dominate—there. Bacteria spend most of their time consuming foods and excreting wastes (much like humans). The wastes from some of those bacteria are sulfur compounds. Sulfur compounds are what ignite the bad-breath brushfire.

The wastes that the bacteria in our mouths excrete are truly some of the most unattractive—and most notorious. That rotten egg smell, technically known as the sulfur compound hydrogen sulfide, is one. The "barnyard" smell, another sulfur compound called methyl mercaptan, is another. These are two of the VSCs, volatile sulfur compounds. The operative word here is *volatile.* These compounds evaporate instantly, and that swiftness allows them to offend everyone around us the minute we open our mouths.

But wait. There's more. Along with the VSCs, oral bacteria also produce other waste products, and each of them smells as nauseating as—or worse than—the VSCs I just described. To name a few of the wastes:

- **Cadaverine:** The name kind of rings a bell, doesn't it? Yup, it's the smell associated with corpses.
- **Putrescine:** Derived from the same Latin word *putre* (which means "to be rotten"), just as the word *putrid* is. The smell? Think of meat once it's past its expiration date.
- **Skatole:** Simply put, it smells like human excrement.

We all have some level of these compounds in our mouths, and in our breath. The good news is that when they're at low levels, they're undetectable to the human nose. The bad news is, when the levels aren't so low, the human nose is the first to find out!

Most of these compounds that cause bad breath are the waste products of anaerobic bacteria. Anaerobic bacteria live under the gum without oxygen. Our mouths experience an ongoing battle for dominance between anaerobic bacteria and aerobic bacteria. It is the precise balance between these two types of bacteria that determines the quality of your breath. Plaque buildup can tip the bacteria scale toward bad breath. So the more plaque that forms on teeth or gums, the more oxygen is depleted, the easier it is for anaerobic bacteria to thrive, and the worse your breath becomes.

Do You Have Bad Breath?

Following is a list of varied telltale signs that could be telling you it's time to supersize the mouthwash.

ROTTEN LUCK

Some people have worse breath than others. Even the most diligent VSC fighter could still possess bad breath. That's because, for reasons that have never been figured out, some of us are just blessed with the ability to produce fewer anaerobic bacteria (and are less likely to have bad breath) than others who produce more (and are more likely to have it), no matter how protein-free their diets may be.

- **Dry mouth:** With less saliva in your mouth, there's less oxygen because saliva contains oxygen, which you need to keep your mouth healthy and fresh. Less oxygen creates an anaerobic environment (it doesn't require oxygen to survive), which encourages sulfur-producing bacteria. These bacteria create the sulfur gases that create bad breath.
- **A white-coated tongue:** A dry mouth provides the perfect home for anaerobic bacteria to be fruitful and multiply, encouraging more sulfur compounds to rise to the tongue's surface. When you have a dry mouth, there's no saliva to flush. It's like a toilet bowl without water.
- **Constantly clearing your throat or having post-nasal drip:** Not only do anaerobic bacteria create bad breath by breaking down protein from food we've eaten, but they also go after the protein in post-nasal drip and mucus, turning that into VSCs as well. The same chemical process happens when you have a sore throat or a cold.

- **Sleeping with your mouth open or snoring:** The constant force of air in and out of the mouth dries it and decreases the amount of saliva.
- **A bad taste in your mouth after drinking milk, coffee, or beer:** When the sugars in these liquids get broken down by the bacteria and turn into acids, you get an acidic, metallic taste in your mouth. Beer contains not only sugars but also carbohydrates, so the bacteria do double duty breaking down both, which leave a particularly bad taste in your mouth.
- **A constant sour, bitter, or metallic taste in your mouth:** Your mouth is a veritable petri dish—drop some sugar in, and it's attacked by those bacteria, then becomes superacidic. If this goes on all the time, it's pretty likely your breath is bad most of the time.
- **Poor oral hygiene:** Lack of flossing allows the anaerobic bacteria to colonize.

Bad-Breath Proponents

While it remains a mystery why some of us have worse breath than others, there are factors that can exacerbate the condition even more. And some are more obvious than others:

- **Thick saliva:** The thicker your saliva, the less oxygen it contains. The less oxygen it contains, the less fresh your mouth—and breath—will be.
- **Smoking:** A top culprit for dry mouth.
- **Alcohol:** Another agent that can promote dry mouth.
- **Prescription medications and anti-histamines:** Both have drying effects on the mouth.

- **Old, worn dental work:** If your old dental work (old composites, old silver fillings, or old crowns) has a rough surface (versus a smooth one), bacteria are more likely to colonize there. The restoration becomes a plaque trap that's impossible to clean. When dentistry is counterproductive—causing more problems and harm to a patient than if it had never been done at all—it's called iatrogenic dentistry. I'd say about 50 to 60 percent of the dentistry that's performed is, unfortunately, iatrogenic.

- **Gastric reflux:** Bad breath can be caused by gastric juices—a problem that's hard to solve, but can be done. Ask your doctor about prescribing a medication to get this condition under control.

You Breathe Out What You Eat

Of course, many different foods encourage bad breath. Some are obvious; others may influence you to change your usual menu selections.

- **High-protein foods:** Bacteria love glomming onto proteins, so high-protein foods contribute generously to halitosis. Top contenders are fish, red meat, and beans.

- **Coffee:** Caffeinated or not, coffee contains high levels of acid, and bacteria love acid as much as they love protein. Acid, however, also causes bacteria to reproduce more rapidly, resulting in a bitter taste in the mouth.

- **Onions and garlic:** Both are packed with odorous molecules that are actually sulfur compounds themselves.
- **Sugar:** Sugar encourages bacteria to reproduce and create even more volatile sulfur compounds. Sugar can attract other bacteria and produce glycan strands with it, which result in thick layers of plaque on tooth enamel and around the gums. This leads to decay and gingivitis, which translates into worse breath.
- **Acidic foods and drinks:** Along with aiding bacteria reproduction, acids are also great at creating sour, bitter, and/or metallic tastes in the mouth.
- **Dairy products:** Lactose intolerance causes more than stomach discomfort. It means the inability to break down the lactose protein that's in dairy foods. This results in a buildup of amino acids, which easily convert into volatile sulfur compounds thanks to the anaerobic bacteria in the tongue.

Take Back Your Breath

The most effective ways to tame bad breath are:

- Have your teeth professionally cleaned at least three times a year.
- Floss every day.
- Brush at least twice a day.
- Brush and scrape your tongue frequently.
- Try an anti-bacterial gel.
- Use an alcohol-free mouthwash once a day.

- Use anti-bacterial sprays. They're also a quick way to give your mouth a clean sweep. Stick one in your purse or leave one by your front door so you'll get into the habit of using it right before you leave the house.

- Drink water frequently, both to keep lingering food particles from sticking as well as to fend off dry mouth.

- Eat right. Choose less acidic food and balance the pH levels in your mouth (more on this in chapter 6).

SELF-AWARENESS TEST

Still not sure whether you're an offender? Here are two simple tests you can give yourself to judge your breath.

- Wipe the surface of your mouth with a piece of cotton gauze and smell that. This is probably the most honest way to judge. Moreover, if you notice a yellowish stain on the cotton, that's a likely sign that you have an elevated sulfide production level.

- Lick the back of your hand. Let it dry for about ten seconds, then smell. If you notice an odor, you have a breath disorder, because the sulfur salts from your tongue have been transferred to your hand.

There. Now you know. In the long run, you'll be glad.

SIX

YOUR MOUTH, YOUR HEALTH

I f you brush, floss, avoid sugar, drag yourself in for a cleaning two or three times a year—how is it you can still end up with nagging issues such as sore gums, sensitive teeth, or even nighttime teeth grinding? The answer is that there's a lot more to oral care than just the basics you were taught in grade school. The state of your mouth affects and is affected by the rest of your body, and there are many simple ways you can target oral problems and maintain the smile you've worked so hard to get.

INTAKE

When you eat right, you know it. You can feel it. Optimum nutrients not only make your body run more

STEVIA: THE ALKALINIZING SWEETENER
THAT STANDS ALONE

Sugar is, plain and simple, the mouth's number one trou-
blemaker. It causes decay, and it promotes plaque. But
substituting artificial sweeteners isn't really a great alternative, either, as they're full of all sorts of unhealthy and
even potentially dangerous ingredients. One alkalinizing
sweetener that's natural, though, is called stevia. Stevia
comes from the stevia plant, which is grown mostly in
South America and parts of Asia, where it's become one
of the most popular low-calorie sweeteners. It is also
used in homeopathic treatments for everything from
hypertension, weight loss, digestion problems, diabetes,
and skin diseases to physical and mental fatigue. Stevia
has even been shown to suppress the growth of bacteria
in the mouth (from a study conducted at Hiroshima University). Gaining quickly in popularity, stevia should be
available at your neighborhood health food store.

efficiently, but they protect your body's cells for the
long haul. This goes for all parts of your body—not
least of all, your mouth. All foods have a pH level. Low-
pH foods have high acid levels (dangerous when abun-
dant); higher-pH foods are the alkalinizing ones (and
better for you). The more acidifying foods you eat, the

SMILE-FRIENDLY FOOD vs. SMILE-CHALLENGING FOOD

FOOD	ALKALINIZING CHOICES	ACIDIFYING CHOICES
Fruits	Most fruits are alkalinizing: apples, apricots, avocados, bananas, cherries, oranges, grapes, peaches, pears, pineapples, strawberries	Blueberries, cranberries, currants, prunes, canned or glazed fruits
Veggies	Beets, broccoli, carrots, celery, eggplant, garlic, green beans, kale, lettuce, mushrooms, onions, peppers, sprouts, squash, tomatoes	Black beans, chickpeas, corn, lentils, lima beans, olives, potatoes, squash, soybeans
Nuts	Almonds, flaxseed, pumpkin seeds	Cashews, peanuts, pecans, walnuts
Proteins	Eggs, chicken breast, tofu, yogurt	Beef, duck, lamb, pork, turkey, basically all fish
Beverages	Fresh and unsweetened fruit juices, regular and herbal teas, vegetable juices, water	All kinds of alcoholic beverages, soda
Seasonings	Apple cider vinegar, chili peppers, cinnamon, curry, garlic, ginger, mustard, salt, all herbs	Ketchup, mustard, mayonnaise pepper and most (all distilled) vinegars, including balsamic
Oils		Just about every type of oil—from olive to canola to sesame—is acidifying
Dairy		All dairy is acidifying
Sweeteners	Stevia	Nearly all sweeteners—both natural and saccharine—are acidifying

more loaded your mouth is with bacteria that cause plaque and decay. The right balance between the two should be a diet majoring in alkalinizing with a minor in acidifiying. The sad truth is that the average American eats mostly acidifying food, with minimal alkalinizing intake. You want to aim for the complete opposite: 75 percent alkalinizing, 25 percent acidifying.

HOLD THE PROTEIN

One of the main reasons that Americans' diets are so highly acidic is the overabundance of protein we eat. Protein fuels the acid in our saliva. It contains tons of sulfur and phosphorus, which turn into sulfuric and phosphoric acids, which then go about their business of demineralizing teeth. As if that weren't enough, protein also lowers white blood cell production, which weakens our immune system. The recommended daily intake of protein is sixty-three grams for males and fifty grams for females, but most Americans eat nearly *twice* that amount. By the same token, we aren't consuming anywhere *near* the amount of fruits and veggies that we're supposed to. By making a conscious effort to swap meat courses for vegetarian options just a few meals a week, you can help create a healthier environment for your teeth and gums to thrive.

In his book *Healthy Mouth, Healthy Body,* holistic dentist Victor Zeines identifies the top ten best foods you can put in your mouth—*for* your mouth.

1. Asparagus.
2. Beets.
3. Broccoli.
4. Carrots.
5. Cauliflower.
6. Celery.
7. Lettuce.
8. Kale.
9. Onions.
10. Spinach.

ORAL HEALTH IS THE PORTAL TO OVERALL HEALTH

When your body's not getting enough proper nutrition, it can show up on your tongue, it can irritate your gums, and it can harbor itself within the roots of your teeth. Very often, when something flares up, loosens, or simply looks different within your mouth, it's your body's way of asking for some type of nutrient it doesn't have enough of.

Use the chart on the following page to match oral health flare-ups with the vitamin and mineral commonly attributed to them. Most abnormal symptoms will disappear soon after a diet is adjusted to include proper nutrients. If symptoms persist, though, do be sure to consult a dentist with your concerns.

ORAL HEALTH FLARE-UPS: NUTRITIONAL SOLUTIONS

AILMENTS OR SYMPTOMS	DEFICIENT VITAMINS OR MINERALS	DR. LEVINE'S RX
Loose teeth, premature tooth loss, softening of teeth, bleeding of gums	Calcium	Milk, yogurt, cheese, tofu, canned sardines or salmon, spinach
Inflamed gum tissue	Magnesium	Halibut, artichokes, spinach, broccoli, green beans, tofu, cashews, sunflower seeds
Shiny red lips, sore tongue, cracks and sores at the corner of the mouth	Vitamin B_2 (riboflavin)	Almonds, broccoli, kale, spinach, lentils, mushrooms, okra, oysters, milk, eggs, sunflower seeds
Red and/or swollen tip of tongue with dry, smooth edges, sores at mouth edges, general mouth pain	Vitamin B_3 (niacin)	Avocados, potatoes, lean ground beef, liver, shrimp
Sore burning mouth, sores at edge of mouth, smooth tongue	Vitamin B_6	Bananas, watermelon, broccoli, spinach, tomato juice, acorn squash, white rice, chicken breast
Bad breath, sores at edge of mouth, bright red tongue that may have fissures, loss of taste, dry mouth, numbness and bleeding	Vitamin B_{12}	Poultry, fish, shellfish, meats, milk, eggs
Bleeding gums, lowered immune response, infections (such as yeast infection) in mouth, impaired taste	Vitamin C or vitamin A	Spinach, broccoli, red bell peppers, snow peas, kiwi, mango, orange, grapefruit juice, strawberries, carrots, kale or other green leafy vegetables, papaya, peaches, red pepper, winter squash
Softening of teeth, increased bleeding, yeast infections	Vitamin D	Egg yolk, fortified milk, liver, fatty fish
Loss of sensation in tongue, loss of taste, dry mouth, susceptibility to gum disease	Zinc	Spinach, green peas, lentils, tomato juice, turkey (dark meat), lean ground beef, lean sirloin steak, plain yogurt, Swiss cheese, ricotta cheese

---

DEAR DENTAL DIARY

If you tend to have oral nuisances, try keeping a food journal, if only for a few days. Jot down everything you eat, then add up the acidifiers and compare them with the alkalinizers. Afterward, check out your mouth to see if your gums are indicative of your diet. If you are diligent about your record keeping, it could very well show you where and how you are making progress.

Should You Detox Your Mouth?

After checking out the acidifying and alkalinizing lists above, then thinking back to what you've eaten this week, you should be able to easily determine whether a mouth detox might do you good. If your mouth is sugared up and overly acidified, a short-term detox can be really helpful—and really healthful. Just a few days of eating only alkalinizing food will help readjust the pH balance in there.

When to Pop the Vitamins

When you don't have the time to eat optimally nutritional foods, or when certain circumstances don't allow it (business trips, wintertime when your grocery store shelves aren't fully stocked with fresh produce), vitamin supplements can fill in for the real thing.

Antioxidants, such as vitamins A, C, and E and

CAUTION: DIETING CAN KILL A SMILE

It's no wonder dieters aren't usually smiling. First of all, depriving a body of adequate amounts of food is never a recipe for happiness. But what's even more disturbing is that crash dieting and yo-yo dieting can do a number on teeth because they make the body more vulnerable to vitamin deficiencies, especially D, B_{12}, and calcium, not to mention certain minerals and proteins that are missing from most diets. Diet pills can also prove detrimental to a smile by drying up the mouth and decreasing the amount of saliva flow. The chemicals in these drugs increase acid levels in the mouth, which leads to tooth decay. This is why so many chronic dieters, and nearly all sufferers of eating disorders, have such poor oral health.

Coenzyme Q10, are excellent for keeping gums healthy. They protect them against cell damage and promote healing in the area as well. Vitamin C, which plays an integral part in collagen production, also makes gum tissue more resistant to bacteria spreading and colonizing there. Vitamin C also promotes healthy capillaries, which help keep the tissue in the mouth healthy. Basically, if your body doesn't have sufficient amounts of vitamin C, your gums could bleed or become swollen; in the worst-case scenario, it could result in tooth loss. Coenzyme Q10 helps protect gums from periodontitis and strengthens the immune system.

PUT SOME MUSCLE IN THAT BITE

One of the most important things you can do for your teeth is strengthen them. Since teeth are vulnerable to de-mineralization when acid levels are high, ideally they should be re-mineralized. Alkalinizing foods and saliva can fortify teeth only to a certain extent. But you can get extra help from nutrients such as calcium, magnesium, and phosphorus—they're especially helpful in re-mineralizing tooth enamel, which strengthens it against plaque. Also, look for toothpastes that have the ability to re-mineralize through ingredients such as calcium and phosphates.

STRESS AND THE SMILE

From infertility to back problems to heart conditions, nowadays we're seeing strong links between high stress levels and a host of health problems. But were you aware that stress can contribute significantly to a number of oral health problems, too?

- **Temporomandibular joint (TMJ) disorder and myofascial pain dysfunction (MPD):** Stress makes our jaw do all kinds of dangerous dances of clenching and grinding. The more tension you have, the more clenching and grinding you do. These types of abnormal jaw positioning often begin as myofascial pain dysfunction and develop into temporomandibular joint disorder, both of which are stress-related. Such disorders begin with jaw tightness, muscle soreness, and pain. If not treated, they can lead to internal displacement, which disrupts the alignment of the disc that separates the lower jaw from the upper jaw (temporomandibular joint). If you clench or grind your teeth, have your dentist fit you for a night guard and evaluate your bite.

- **Viral infection:** Such infection is a direct result of a depressed immune response, in which stress often plays a role.

- **Aphthous ulcers (canker sores):** There are different theories about what triggers aphthous ulcers, more commonly known as canker sores. The fact of the matter is that there are many: depressed immune response, improper nutrition, trauma from dental work. But the one thing these culprits have in common is that they're all stress-induced in one way or another. If you find yourself getting one canker sore after another, crank up your supply of vitamin B_{12}, avoid hot foods, and ask your dentist to prescribe a topical cream to ease the condition.

- **Type 1 herpes lesions:** Another condition that stems from a depressed immune response, herpes lesions appear on the gingival area. Again, lowering your stress levels will greatly help.

Stress and Cortisol

While endorphins are fairly easy to release, cortisol, known as the king of stress hormones, has a tendency to stick in humans and stay there, which causes all sorts of health problems. Built-up cortisol can cause weight gain, depression, osteoporosis, even heart disease and cancer. Animals secrete cortisol automatically as part of their innate survival skills. When they sense danger, their brain alerts their adrenal glands to secrete adrenaline and cortisol, which help fuel their fight-or-flight response. Now, if only humans could automatically kick into "fight or flight" as instinctively as animals in the wild do, we'd be much better off. When *we* get hit with daily stresses (work deadlines; nagging bosses, spouses, or children; bills), we usually don't fight *or* flight our way out of them. Unfortunately, we instead retain cortisol, and thus internalize stress.

Despite the resistance and/or inability to release cortisol, you can certainly lower its levels by making some minor adjustments:

- Get more sleep—a minimum of seven hours and forty minutes per day.
- Eat a better balanced diet.
- Stay away from supplements that increase cortisol levels, such as ephedra, guaraná, yohimbe, and caffeine.
- Take a daily multivitamin that has calcium, magnesium, vitamin C, and B-complex vitamins—they're needed for a proper stress response.
- Consider taking a cortisol-controlling supplement containing omega-3 fatty acids.

TRANSLATING TONGUES

The tongue is a great indicator of overall health. You know how the bottoms of feet are known as the body's map in the Eastern practice of reflexology? Well, the tongue is even more telling, and its signs are a lot easier to read for detecting imbalances in your body.

THE TONGUE IS TELLING

IF YOUR TONGUE IS . . .	IT MEANS THAT YOU COULD . . .
. . . yellowish or yellow-green	. . . have liver or gallbladder problems
. . . gray or brownish gray	. . . have stomach or intestinal problems
. . . white	. . . be releasing toxins
. . . white with a reddish border	. . . have a toxic colon
. . . covered with a cracked coating of white	. . . have digestive disorders
. . . coated with red spots on the tip	. . . have heart problems
. . . turning from white to yellow at the root	. . . have kidney problems
. . . indented or cracked on the surface	. . . probably have a vitamin deficiency
. . . outlined with tooth marks on its edges	. . . have a mineral deficiency

Tongue Cleansing

You can help get both your tongue and the rest of your body back in balance with a body-cleansing diet, just for one day.

- **Breakfast:** Grapefruit or other fresh fruit *or* vegetable juice.

- **Midmorning snack:** Sprouts with tomatoes, onion, or avocado.
- **Lunch:** Fresh fruit or vegetable salad with cold-press oil and lemons or herbs as dressing.
- **Midafternoon snack:** More sprouts.
- **Dinner:** Salad or a plate of baked or steamed vegetables.

Following this menu for even one day will help the body detoxify and cleanse your system.

ORAL CANCER SELF-EXAM

Oral cancer affects about thirty thousand Americans each year, and only half of those diagnosed live for five more years. As with most cancers, early detection is key, and self-exams are quick and fairly simple since the symptoms are easy to spot. They may include:

- A lump in the throat.
- A thickening or lump(s) in the lining of the mouth.
- Tongue numbness.
- Red or white lesions in the mouth.
- Any dark blue or black spots on the tongue.

Once a week, give yourself a little "Ah" in front of the mirror and check out your tongue (top and bottom), your gum areas, the back of your mouth, and the inside cheek areas of your mouth. Being on the lookout for any abnormal activity in the mouth can help you stay on top of your own health. But you can't be your own dentist. See your dentist or dental hygienist every six months. If you've had significant dental work done, schedule appointments more frequently, such as every three or four months.

SEVEN

MOUTH BREAKDOWNS— & BREAKTHROUGHS

What does it mean when teeth fall out in a dream? The answers vary. The armchair Freud chalks it up to sexual inadequacy. Other dream interpreters say it's a sign of being out of control or overburdened. Most, though, say that it's connected to public exposure, the fear of exposing yourself to others in an uncomfortable way. Finally, some interpret it as the simple fear of losing your teeth.

Smiles have some worthy enemies to be reckoned with. Despite the constant advancements in dentistry, there are still plenty of oral headaches that can crop up. Gums bleed. Cavities appear. Tartar builds up. Enamel chips off. Smiles look old. Next, you'll find the various reasons behind the pain, and what can be done to ease it.

PLAQUE AND FORCE

Plaque is what happens when bacteria colonize on a tooth. If food particles stay on or between teeth, and the bacteria is not removed on a daily basis, a natural petri dish forms there. The sugars feed the plaque and encourage it to grow even more. If the bacteria aren't brushed away but linger, this then produces acids, which eventually begin to dissolve the tooth, starting with the enamel.

So the more sugar you eat, the greater the amount of acid is produced in your mouth, and the faster a tooth can dissolve, or de-mineralize, as it's called. The area between the teeth is most vulnerable, since it's the hardest to clean. If the acid isn't cleaned out from there (in other words, if you don't floss), it collects there and burrows a hole into the tooth. This is decay.

Decay is very goal-oriented: Its focus is to destroy a tooth. How? By blasting through that tooth, layer by layer. It starts at the top with the enamel and works its way inward. If it reaches as deeply as the pulp, which is where the tooth's nerve lives, that's when it hurts so badly that it can wake you up faster than any nightmare.

Growing Pains

The pain we get inside our mouths evolves as we get older, just like the rest of our bodies. During our childhood and teen years, we're stuffing ourselves with sugar, so the bacteria are in pig heaven. That's why fluoride is so important then—along with, of course, good oral hygiene and smart nutrition. All these factors help minimize decay. As we get older, our diet changes (less candy), so the bacteria change from aerobic bacteria to the anaerobes that cause gum disease.

There are two types of bacteria. Aerobic bacteria live with oxygen, love the company of food particles in the mouth, and feed on sugar. Anaerobic bacteria exist without oxygen and feed off dead skin cells and other bacteria. Both need to exist in your mouth, but when your oral environment gets out of balance, that's when the trouble starts. Anaerobic bacteria not only are responsible for creating bad breath but also create plaque, which leads to inflammation in the gums, which leads to both tooth loss and bone loss. And this is what we call periodontal disease.

Force

Force can break down a smile's structure because it wears down the teeth and encourages gums to recede. That gum recession leads to an exposed root, which is dangerous and can be really painful. Imagine a wire that's lost its protective insulation. The wire becomes both precarious and sensitive, and it's no different with your gums. When a root gets exposed like this, there are projections called dentinal tubules, which send an impulse to the nerve of the tooth telling your brain to experience pain. It also tells your brain that it had better remove that cold or sweet object from the tooth immediately.

Oral force occurs in many different ways:

- Clenching and grinding—pathological force (harmful).
- Aggressive toothbrushing—pathological force (harmful).
- Hit by a foreign object—random and uncontrolled force (harmful).
- Orthodontics—controlled and directed force (harmless).

While orthodontia is a guided force, teeth weren't made for the other forces, which are either pathological or just plain random and out of control. Forces like these can cause tremendous wear to the top third of the teeth, exposing dentin under the enamel, causing gums to recede, and even creating notches in the root of the tooth, which are called abfractive lesions. Abfractive lesions can begin to form in people as early as their twenties, and the exposed root that results is sensitive to just about everything—cold, heat, sweetness, air.

TOOTH SENSITIVITIES: EVERYBODY HURTS SOMETIMES

Just about everyone experiences some type of tooth sensitivity at one time or another. I'd venture to guess that as many as one in two people have some kind of sensitivity issue with their teeth. Probably more. It can be caused by a number of factors, including:

- Gum recession or decay, both of which can lead to periodontal disease and tooth loss. And teeth are mighty sensitive by that point.
- Physical forces, such as clenching and grinding or overaggressive toothbrush abrasion, either from your own force or from a brush with bristles that are too hard.

Not only can tooth sensitivity be quite painful, it's almost always a warning signal of some kind of problem beginning or growing that could potentially lead to some pretty serious conditions.

The Levels of Tooth Sensitivities

You may have experienced firsthand that there are different kinds of tooth sensitivities. While your teeth may freak out when you bite into a scoop of ice cream, your friend's may tingle when she takes a sip of hot tea. In total, there are four levels of tooth sensitivities. The least serious kind is the one that's sensitive to sweetness, but it can swiftly progress to a biting sensitivity, and that's the most distressing kind. The goal is to catch—and relieve—the sensitivity before it reaches the biting stage.

Of course, within each of the sensitivities are varying degrees of magnitude: Just how cold, how hot, how biting, or how sensitive is the sensation? The more intense it feels, of course, the closer you're inching toward the next level.

1. Sweet Sensitivity

The experience: When something sugary goes in your mouth, you feel an immediate painful response to it. And, when it's removed, the pain disappears just as quickly.

The causes: It could be caused by early decay in the tooth, or it could signal some root exposure (from the gum having receded off the root, leaving its surface exposed).

Worry level: Not too high. Sweet sensitivity is the precursor to all the other sensitivities. If your teeth can't handle biting into a candy bar but are just fine with ice cream and hot chocolate, consider yourself lucky, but also consider having your dentist check the area out.

Treatment: Usually a professional checkup and good cleaning clears up the problem.

2. Cold Sensitivity

The experience: When anything cold goes in your mouth, there's an immediate pain response.

The causes: The decay is either starting to progress a bit farther, or the root exposure has become more significant. If you have old dental work in your mouth (*old* meaning ten years or more), decay could be lurking under an old restoration, making the tooth more sensitive as it edges closer to the nerve. When the nerve gets inflamed, the pulp of the tooth is inflamed as well, and the condition is called reversible pulpitis.

Worry level: These conditions aren't past repair. With the reversible pulpitis condition, the operative word is *reversible.* The nerve is still alive. The tooth can be reinsulated.

Treatment: Reversible pulpitis can be fixed with some type of restoration, such as a bonded filling, inlay/onlay, or crown that seals the tooth well.

3. Heat Sensitivity

The experience: An immediate pain response when eating anything hot.

Causes: Sensitivity to hot temperatures is often coupled with sensitivity to cold temperatures. They are usually caused by the same things: significant decay, root exposure, gum inflammation, and/or reversible pulpitis.

Worry level: Significant. If you're sensitive to heat, the nerve has probably become irreversibly inflamed, and that's irreversible pulpitis. It can't be fixed, and it's on its way to dying.

Treatment: You have two choices: a root canal or tooth extraction. If caught in time, this problem can be remedied by a root canal. However, if you wait too long, and inflammation swells in the bone, the condition could end up being much more painful and warrant tooth extraction. If you experience significant sensitivity to heat in one or more of your teeth, see your dentist immediately.

4. Biting Sensitivity

The experience: Anytime you bite into anything, it hurts. It can get so bad that it can wake you in the middle of the night, writhing in pain.

Causes: There are many causes for biting sensitivity.

Cause #1, Endodontic lesions: These occur when the nerve dies; its dying nerve tissue (called necrotic debris) starts to leak out from the root. This sets off what's called an inflammatory response because the body sees the debris as a foreign invader. This prompts blood to flow into the bone, but it can't expand because it's inelastic, so all this pressure makes it painful.

Worry level: Significant. Your nerve tissue has died. And now the inflammatory response has made the area more painful.

Treatment: Endodontic lesions should be treated by an endodontist (someone who specializes in root canals), who will remove the necrotic debris and seal the end of the root with an inert material. *Inert* means that it's neutral, responds to nothing, and nothing goes through it anymore.

Cause #2, Inner cracks: When an area within the crown of the tooth has cracked, impulses cause fluids to flow through the crack down to the nerve of the tooth, which signals it to respond in pain.

Worry level: The seriousness of this condition varies, depending on the size of the crack within the tooth.

Treatment: It depends on the level of seriousness. In some cases, you can support the tooth all the way around with a crown so that the crack doesn't extend any farther. The crown binds a tooth like the metal reinforcement bands bind a barrel, and it could be made of ceramic, porcelain, or a metal structure. If the fracture is near the gum line, sometimes lowering the gum line through surgery can save it. The worst-case scenario is when the fracture has gone through the tooth down to the root area. When that happens, the tooth needs to be extracted.

Cause #3, Flexure: Flexing happens when decay in or under an old restoration (or filling) eats away at the tooth, destabilizing the tooth, leaving it unsupported, and thus flexing it. And when the tooth flexes, it sends an impulse back to the nerve, and then to the brain, communicating pain.

Worry level: Moderate. This condition can be treated effectively by a dentist. If you think you have flexure, make an appointment within the month.

Treatment: The decay needs to be cleaned out, then the tooth needs to be insulated from inside. If the decay has reached the nerve, both a root canal and then a crown are probably necessary. If the decay hasn't yet reached the nerve, a ceramic or gold restoration can be applied to bring support back to the tooth.

Cause #4, Ligament pain: If a tooth is traumatized, the ligament around the tooth becomes wider, increasing the mobility and causing an inflammation in its ligament space, called ligament pain. Unlike orthodontia, where the force that's applied is measured, an untold, pathological force can cause bone destruction.

Ligament pain can also happen if food (even something as small as a poppy seed) becomes impacted within this ligament somewhere (this is also called a foreign body reaction). Ligament pain can be very subtle, though, and many dentists misdiagnose it for pain from decay in the tooth because you can experience cold and sweet sensitivity.

Treatment: Sometimes the impacted food particle can be flushed out with a rinse. However, more stubborn particles must be removed by a dentist.

ENAMEL AND ITS VULNERABILITIES

Enamel can be attacked a number of ways.

Stress Fractures

The grinding and clenching brought on by high stress levels can encourage the enamel to pop right off a tooth. An exorbitant amount of friction can debilitate a canine, so its neighboring premolars have to fill in. This double workload pushes them in the wrong direction. But they're not made to be moved the way canines can, and when they're pushed too far, the enamel begins to pop off at the gum line. It's like a ceramic rod being bent at both ends. The result is an abfractive lesion at the gum line, which looks like a V-shaped nick in a tree.

Treatment: Canine guidance is restored when the prosthodontist or restorative dentist adds material to the canines, allowing them to separate the teeth behind it. To prevent it from reoccurring, have your dentist make you a night guard.

Stripping from Erosion

Any de-mineralizing agent can cause erosion to the enamel. When tooth whiteners are overused, their chemicals, such as hydrogen peroxide or carbamide peroxide, can eat away at the enamel. An overly acidic diet (sometimes caused by drinking too much orange juice or sucking on lemons) can also contribute to enamel erosion. Of course, this kind of erosion isn't something you can necessarily feel, but your dentist or hygienist will be able to tell.

Treatment: Your dentist or hygienist can provide you with some kind of re-mineralizing therapy.

Stripping from Gastric Juices

Whether they come up of their own accord (as in acid reflux) or with some assistance from you (as in bulimia nervosa), gastric acids erode enamel. Sadly, most dentists can spot bulimics quite easily by the condition of the enamel on their teeth. One of the many side effects of bulimia nervosa is that hydrochloric acid enters the mouth too often, washing away enamel surfaces, and if it continues in a constant manner, teeth will completely lose their enamel.

Treatment: If you suffer from acid reflux, you can try over-the-counter medications or ask your doctor to prescribe a medication. You've probably heard of some gastric reflux medications from their commercials, such as Maalox, Gaviscon, and Prilosec. Of course, anyone suffering from bulimia should seek professional help.

Let Your Dentist Be Your Second Opinion

To determine the cause and severity of tooth sensitivity, dental experts do what is called a differential diagnosis. They examine the presented sensitivity symptoms, then go down a decision tree to determine the cause. A digital X-ray is taken, as well as transillumination of the tooth to detect cracks (with a device called a DIFOTI machine, which can actually detect decay under a restoration), a percussion test (biting test), and an electric pulp test for vitality of the tooth. After that, the clinical exam is done, and by then the problem can usually be narrowed down to one cause.

Oral Fixations Are More Than Just Embarrassing

Has it ever occurred to you that most nervous habits manifest themselves in the mouth? Think about it: nail biting, smoking, teeth grinding. We truly are an oral-fixated species. Too bad, since our mouths aren't really the best places to take out our frustrations. What may be alleviating the stress elsewhere just redirects onto our mouths. So many mouth- and teeth-related habits—some of which we're not even conscious of while we're doing them—can affect your smile, in very bad ways.

Ask yourself. Do you ever . . .

- **. . . brush or floss too aggressively?** If you brush your teeth as though you're trying to scrape their enamel off, you very well might be. Likewise, aggressive flossing can do damage to the gum line.

- **. . . chew the insides of your cheeks?** Not only does this habit cause soreness and those unattractive white spots (medical name: hyperkeratotic lesions), but holding your teeth and jaw in that position traumatizes the joint as well. And that could ultimately shift your teeth's relaxed normal bite.

- **. . . chew on ice?** Biting ice can cause fractures, crack teeth, and break tooth edges. On top of that, artificial surfaces can't hold up against hard ice either, so this habit could destroy a pretty hefty dental investment of bonding and veneers.

- **. . . bite your nails?** Nail biting can chip and crack the edges of teeth, particularly the thin edges.

- **. . . chew on pencils and pens?** Even nonaggressive chewing on objects such as pens, pencils, eyeglasses, hair clips, or pins can crack and fracture tooth edges and break veneers and bonding.

- **. . . crack open nuts with your teeth?** Beware! This habit is even worse than chewing on pens and other objects!

- **. . . tear things open with your teeth?** Do this enough and you'll begin to crack the edges of your teeth.

- **. . . smoke?** Stains! Gum soreness! Gum inflammation! Dry mouth! Damage to the tongue! Bad breath! These are just some of the ways your mouth will suffer if you smoke.

- **. . . use toothpicks to clean out your teeth?** While toothpicks, as well as other cleaning devices, can be effective in cleaning the sulcus area (those V's between your teeth and gums), they can flatten out and/or push up the soft tissue above the teeth and encourage dark triangles to form. Floss or oral irrigators are better alternatives for removing food particles.

- **. . . grind them together?** Clenching and grinding can cause myriad problems. Teeth can crack, veneers can pop off, and this overall wear and tear of teeth's edges—as well as their enamel—can cause major damage over time. After a few years of clenching or grinding, the teeth lose their edges as well as their precision and proper function, causing greater force to the teeth. If you notice the beginning of wear on your front teeth, have your dentist take a look before the problem becomes more serious.

Curbing the Sensitivity

If you're beginning to experience sensitivity, you can try an over-the-counter desensitizing toothpaste, such as Sensodyne or GoSMILE's AM and PM toothpastes. They both use high levels of fluoride mixed with high levels of potassium nitrate (5 percent). However, if the problem persists after about three or four weeks, consult your dentist.

SELF-DIAGNOSIS

It goes without saying that if something feels wrong, like a weird bite, tooth sensitivity, or jaw pain, you should head to the dentist for a professional opinion. But here's a quick tip sheet to look over first. It will help you speak to your dentist about what you think is wrong.

SELF-DIAGNOSIS AT A GLANCE

PROBLEM	WHAT IT LOOKS LIKE	SYMPTOMS	CAUSES	TREATMENT OPTIONS
Decay	Dark spot on top surface or shadow on front of tooth	Starts out as sweet sensitivity progressing to cold, then hot, then ultimately biting and excruciating pain	Improper oral hygiene and too much sugar in diet	Thorough cleaning; restorative dentistry; possible root canal therapy
Uneven bite	Not really visible, but you feel it every time you bite	Discomfort in biting position; soreness in jaw; noise in joint when opening and closing	Growth and development problems; previously done orthodontics; imprecise restorative dentistry; constant clenching and grinding	Orthodontia; bite adjustment (occlusal adjustment); restorative dentistry to reestablish bite
Grinding and clenching	Wear on front teeth; shortened teeth	V-shaped notches in root area; abfractions; cold and sweet sensitivities	Stress-induced clenching and grinding	Restorative dentistry: sealing neck of tooth up from abfraction; adding length to tooth; orthotic night guard to prevent against further wear
Jaw pain: including both TMJ (temporomandibular joint) disorder and/or MPD (myofascial pain dysfunction)	Limited jaw opening; short, worn-down teeth	Muscle soreness, headaches, joint pain, joint noise (clicking or popping in joint area)	Stress-induced grinding or clenching of teeth; poor dentistry	Bite adjustment plus night guard; restorative dentistry; corrective surgery *(continued)*

SELF-DIAGNOSIS AT A GLANCE (continued)

Problem	What it looks like	Symptoms	Causes	Treatment Options
De-mineralization of tooth surfaces	Shortened front teeth; abnormal bite	Sensitivity to sweetness, cold, and hot; pain when biting	Eating disorder (bulimia); overly acidic diet	Removal of causative agent; professional treatment
Receding gums	Gums start to rise off roots, exposing root surfaces	Sweet, cold sensitivity	Heredity; biting stresses; aggressive toothbrushing	Sealing exposed root surface with free gingival graft or restorative dentistry

EIGHT

GUMS BEHAVING BADLY

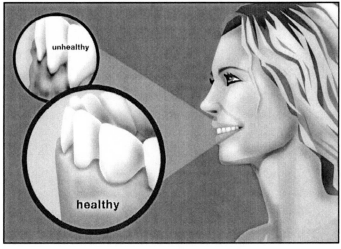

fig. 8.1

A healthy set of gums should be pink and stippled, very tight and bound down. They should have little indents in them like a good set of abs. Those indents signify a certain amount of health. Consider your gums' relationship to your teeth to be like skin over bones. If you don't nurture them with proper flossing and brushing, they will eventually turn on you. Gums do not take kindly to neglect.

123

According to the American Academy of Periodontology, more than 75 percent of adults over the age of thirty-five have some form of periodontal disease. That includes gingivitis and bone loss. By now you know that if you let either of these conditions go untreated, you can end up losing your teeth.

In fact, by neglecting your gums, you could end up losing a lot more than your teeth. A mouth with diseased gums can set off influential amounts of bacterial pro-inflammatory components into the bloodstream, which can travel to any vital organ and cause serious inflammation there as well. Your red, swollen gums could ultimately give you heart disease. For these reasons, periodontal disease is becoming known as systemic periodontal disease.

GINGIVITIS

Diseased gums are easy to spot—they're red, they're inflamed. If yours are red around the area where your tooth meets the gum—if that area is sensitive to the touch, or if it bleeds when you brush or floss—you've most likely got some degree of gingivitis.

Here's how it happens: Bleeding, sensitive gums are usually signs that plaque is hiding somewhere in the area, probably within the gum's pocket, that deepened furrow between the neck of the tooth and the gum. A pocket is a sulcus that's become too deep, and the

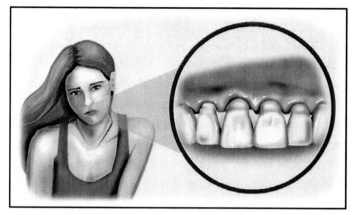

fig. 8.2

deeper the space, the more difficult it is for both you and even your dental expert to reach. So, since cleaning it is impossible, plaque can pile up with no disturbances from a toothbrush, floss, or any at-home tool. After a while, the plaque hardens, and it must be removed.

This plaque is a different kind of plaque from the one that de-mineralizes a tooth. This plaque is formed from the anaerobic bacteria mentioned earlier. When these bacteria accumulate around the gum area on the root surface, the gum becomes inflamed, sort of like a splinter that's lodged itself under skin. This is another example of an inflammatory response. And this is a crucial time. If you don't take care of this inflammation, you'll soon find yourself crossing over from gingivitis to the much darker world of periodontal disease and bone loss.

PERIODONTAL DISEASE

While gum disease is very visible, periodontal disease is not. It's usually painless at the beginning, but it can worsen and become quite serious without you even reealizing it. Like gum inflammation, bone destruction can be intercepted by your dentist. If the disease hasn't reached severe levels, a treatment called phase one perio, also known as soft tissue management, can be effective in stopping bone destruction.

Phase one perio involves a lot of scraping, digging, and smoothing of the diseased root surface in the diseased gum. Called scaling and root planing, it's a nonsurgical treatment that involves removing the offending substance above and below the gum.

Scaling removes the deposits of tartar above and below the gum. A scaler looks like a pen with a curved

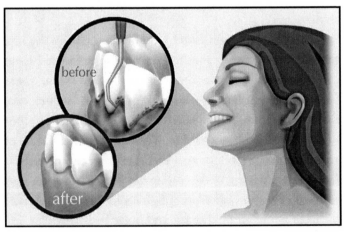

fig. 8.3

end, making it easier for the dentist to get into the hard-to-reach spots, such as the pockets. Scaling also removes any diseased bacteria (called bacterial endo-toxins) that may have gotten under the gum and stuck to the root surfaces. After scaling, most hygienists go over the area again with an ultrasonic vibrating tool, which acts like a mini sandblaster that literally blasts the more accessible hardened deposits off the teeth.

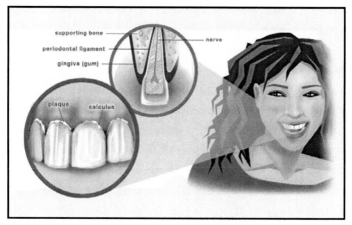

fig. 8.4

Root planing goes after the bacterial endotoxins *under* the gum and removes any diseased cementum (that cell layer covering the outside of the root that keeps the tooth attached) that might be there as well. Root planing smooths the area the same way a car-penter buffs away roughness in a piece of wood.

If the gum tissue is also inflamed, the hygienist or dentist will also do something called curettage. Curettage removes the inner lining of the inflamed tissue, which then allows the new tissue to heal against the newly cleaned, "buffed" root surface.

Once cleaned out, the gum tissue should shrink and tighten around the newly cleaned root surface, eliminating much of the pocket. Once the tissue is healed, the pocket then has to be monitored to see if phase one was successful.

Before he sends you home to care for your tender healing gums, your dentist may also insert a chemotherapeutic agent into the area, either in a chip that he'll stick under your gum flap or a gel, called Arrestin, which he'll insert with a syringe. They usually contain an antibiotic, such as doxycycline or minocycline, which kills any remaining bacteria, speeds healing time, and helps the pocket shrink faster. They're time-released and continue to work for about ten days. Many dentists also like to give patients an anti-bacterial rinse called Peridex (lab name: chlorhexidine gluconate). Peridex stains teeth, so you need to overcompensate with an at-home stain-removing, whitening product during the entire time that you use it.

Phase Two Perio-Flap Surgery

If the scaling and root planing and curettage aren't enough, the pockets have to then be surgically removed. This procedure is done by a periodontist, who specializes in the supporting structures of the teeth, gum, and bone. Flap surgery removes the excess soft tissue and shapes the underlying bone so that the pocket will heal back to a less deep, healthy sulcus. Afterward, the gums get sutured back into place, so the tissue fits tightly around the tooth again.

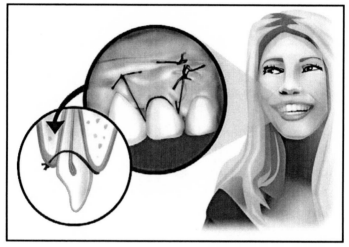

fig. 8.5

Flap surgery allows the periodontist to visualize the bone, so he can then either take away bone to remove the defect (which is the pocket) or graft new bone into the defect—in effect, adding to it. It all depends on the anatomy of the particular defect.

Bone and Tissue Grafting

Like skin grafting, bone and tissue grafting encourages regrowth. The technique is called tissue regeneration; it involves a small piece of meshed fabric that gets placed between the bone and gum tissue. Tissue regeneration also helps prevent the gum tissue from growing into the area where the bone should be growing, so both can grow back in peace.

OTHER CAUSES OF GUM CONDITIONS

Aside from plaque, other conditions can trigger red and bleeding gums:

- **Pregnancy:** Those hormonal changes that can cause strange food cravings and unexplained bouts of tears can also cause gums to bleed. There's even a name for this condition—pregnancy gingivitis. Hormonal changes cause an increased sensitivity to plaque, causing increased inflammation. The good news is that the inflammation can be monitored closely by your dental team pros, along with, of course, meticulous home care.
- **A challenged immune system:** Your gums might bleed more when your immune system is burdened, such as when you have a cold. That's because the mouth picks up viruses more easily when the immune system is down, causing gums to be more swollen and sensitive.
- **Stress:** While our bodies are used to the usual expected levels of stress, excessive amounts can be too much, and the body's stress can overload the mouth. Finding alternative ways to alleviate stress should return the gums to normal.

- **Heredity:** A study in the *Journal of Medical Genetics* indicated that gum disease could be a genetic predisposition. Researchers discovered that changes in a gene for the enzyme cathepsin C are responsible for a condition known as Papillon-Lefèvre syndrome. Along with scaly and warty skin thickening and an erosion of the soft tissues that line the mouth and connecting gums, another symptom is inflamed gums.

- **Juvenile periodontosis:** As its name suggests, juvenile periodontosis affects young people, specifically those who have a virulent type of bacteria that's hard to stop and treat successfully. In many cases, these patients can lose their first molars and front teeth if aggressive periodontal therapy isn't performed. Fortunately, there are microbiological techniques that can isolate the bacteria to make this disease easier for periodontists to diagnose and treat. Treatment involves a microbiological and surgical approach, which, along with meticulous home care, often cures this condition.

Occasional bleeding is common in gums, especially if you're just starting out on a disciplined flossing regime. But the bleeding should dissipate within a week. If it doesn't, and you've already had any plaque properly removed by your dental hygienist, it is urgent that you see a dentist. Sometimes bleeding gums are signals of something much more serious, such as a blood disorder or even leukemia. When the puffiness isn't related to a plaque issue, a blood test should determine whether there is another health issue.

DOS AND DON'TS FOR HEALTHY GUMS

Do brush and floss teeth at least twice a day. Carry a hygienically protected toothbrush (in a toothbrush case) and floss with you.

Don't go overboard with sugared and fatty foods.

Do take calcium and vitamin C—both promote healthy gums. New supplements are being introduced to the American market that will help soft tissue healing and improve health. Learn more about these supplements in the final chapter, New Frontiers.

Don't stress out. Your gums are just one in a long list of parts of your body that suffer from too much stress.

Do get your teeth professionally cleaned at least twice a year—more if your gums look inflamed or if you've had significant dentistry in the past. (Restorative dentistry is especially prone to breaking down, because the artificial surface is like a magnet to plaque—much more so than a natural surface.)

Do eat foods high in fiber, such as fruits and vegetables, which fortify both the hard and soft tissues of the mouth.

NINE

THE WHITENING STORM

Today *everyone* wants a brighter, whiter smile. And what began as something only a handful of dentists were experimenting with has become a standard procedure for most. Nearly all dentists now offer whitening treatments in their offices. There are even whitening franchises, such as BriteSmile. High-end markets, including spas, beauty boutiques, and prestige department stores, carry smile whiteners, and the number of at-home whitening kits on drugstore shelves is starting to edge out toothpastes in the battle for retail space.

Currently, one hundred million Americans whiten their teeth. Of those, ten million will go to their dentists for these services. And it is estimated that the market for tooth-whitening products and services will reach fifteen billion dollars by the year 2010.

That's a remarkable amount of business for an industry that hardly existed as recently as five years ago.

According to the American Academy of Cosmetic Dentistry, the number of whitening and bleaching procedures has increased more than 300 percent in the past five years. Between the in-office procedures and the at-home systems, tooth whitening is now a six-hundred-million-dollar-a-year industry, and it shows no signs of leveling off anytime soon.

This chapter is devoted to helping you achieve a brighter, whiter smile. Whether it's performed in a dentist's office or on your own with one of the various dental-administered or over-the-counter products, there's a wide range of whitening options to choose from. Throughout each section, I'll cover costs, the results you can expect, and how easy or difficult it will be to get these results. Use this chapter as a guide to help you find which whitening path (if any) is the one for you. First, though, it's important to understand what other factors affect the color of your teeth.

THE MANY SHADES OF WHITE

The outermost section of the tooth is the enamel, and beneath it is the dentin. The enamel lies over the dentin like frosted glass, and the tooth color is reflected from that underlying dentin layer.

Even if we never smoked or drank red wine and avoided staining foods altogether, we *still* wouldn't share the same tooth color. Original tooth shades are genetically predetermined. However, dozens of factors influence these shades.

Along with genetics, color-influencing factors can be congenital, metabolic, chemical, infectious, and environmental. If any of these factors came in contact with your teeth before you reached the age of eight or nine, the chances of your teeth being affected in some way were higher because they were still forming at that point, so they were far more vulnerable to outside disturbances. These childhood "disturbances" range from having taken medications such as tetracycline to having high fevers, exposure to excessive amounts of fluoride (whether from water, fluoride supplements, or even overzealous use of rinses and toothpastes), and inadequate oral hygiene.

Not All Stains Are the Same

There are two different levels of stains: intrinsic and extrinsic.

- **Intrinsic staining** is the result of all those varied influences that might occur during the tooth's formative years. Intrinsic staining also includes the yellowing of teeth that happens *later* in life, as we age. Along with wrinkled skin, sore backs, and compromised eyesight, teeth just naturally yellow as we get older and the color-producing dentin layer thickens with age. Intrinsic stains are much more difficult to remove.
- **Extrinsic staining** happens when highly pigmented foods linger on the tooth for a lengthy period of time and ultimately find their way into the superficial layers of the enamel. These stains are much easier to

WHEN YOU EAT STAINING FOODS . . .

- Have a glass of water nearby when you're drinking wine or coffee. After every few sips, take some water and swish it around in your mouth. That will help keep the staining pigments from lingering.
- Whenever possible, brush your teeth soon after a meal if any of its components was staining.
- Give extra attention to the areas between your teeth; that's where stains tend to secure themselves and build up over time.
- Never skip bedtime brushing after a staining meal. You've already allowed ample time for the pigments to make themselves at home. Waiting until the next morning is as good as putting a finishing topcoat over the stains.

manage than the intrinsic ones, and simply becoming aware of when you're eating or drinking staining foods is a great first step.

The Worst Offenders

You probably already know what the highly pigmented staining culprits are: red wine, coffee, and tea. But there are others that might not be as obvious, yet they're just as staining. These include blueberries, soy sauce, balsamic vinegar, tomato sauce, and certain fruit juices (grape and cranberry).

CERTAIN FOODS CAN *HELP* WHITEN TEETH

The good news is that along with being generally good for you, certain fruits and vegetables come equipped with smile-maintaining and smile-protecting powers. Foods that require a lot of chewing, such as apples, celery, and carrots, whiten teeth naturally because they're like stain exfoliants. You know how great your skin looks and feels after you've used a facial scrub? These foods perform the same kind of sloughing action on teeth, helping to keep them clear of clingy stains. Greens such as spinach, broccoli, and lettuce also prevent staining because they create a film over teeth that actually acts as a barrier. So be sure to order a side of spinach the next time you're enjoying that fine glass of Bordeaux at your favorite restaurant.

THE WHITENING CONCEPT IS BORN

As long as there have been staining foods and tobacco, there has been the desire for a whiter smile. Even centuries ago, when just managing to hold on to your own teeth was a talent, a whiter smile was still the dental Holy Grail. It goes as far back as the seventeenth century.

Multitasking was pervasive then, so the duties of dentistry fell upon the village barber. Of course, this was long before drills and fillings were around, so the barber's dental care consisted mostly of yanking out decayed teeth. Occasionally, though, the barber would file teeth down, then coat them with nitric acid. While that acid did in fact bring about a wonderful white hue to teeth, it was also highly corrosive, so the magic didn't last very long. That short-term "whitener" also caused tremendous destruction to the tooth enamel, eventually causing huge amounts of decay. Fortunately, nitric acid has gone the way of the gallows, and teeth can now be whitened without danger, pain, acid, or barber.

Choose Your Whitening Method

Like hair coloring or perms, the success of whitening is all about the concentration of the active ingredients and the amount of time those actives are, in fact, active on the teeth. This holds true for every type of whitening, from professional to at-home brands. But both the active ingredients and the way in which they're applied vary.

Whitening 101

It's pretty simple chemistry. Teeth are whitened by hydrogen peroxide. When the hydrogen peroxide touches the tooth, a type of oxygen, called free radical oxygen, gets "excited," meaning that it revs up and dives through the tooth's enamel to its dentin, which is where the stains live. The oxygen hits the stains, breaks them up, and wipes them off.

Both in-office whitening and out-of-office whitening

(be it an ampoule, strip, brush-on gel, or tray-and-gel system) use oxygen to penetrate the dentin. However, during office procedures, a high-intensity light activates the oxygen to reach the dentin and wipe away the stains. The light-on-peroxide activation lasts about twenty minutes and is repeated about three or four times in one sitting.

Over-the-counter products, however, have no special light. They rely instead on contact time. When the peroxide comes in contact with saliva, the oxygen flies out and does its stuff. These formulas contain only a fraction of the hydrogen peroxide that the in-office ones do (6 percent versus 20 percent or higher) so they can stay on teeth for longer periods of time. But these aren't a one-shot deal. Most over-the-counter companies suggest ten days to two weeks of daily use of the product for about an hour or so per day. Recent studies have shown that repetitive whitening at safe, low concentrations of the active ingredients gives longer lasting results.

There are a number of caveats about each of the different whitening treatments, but I'll get into them later on in the chapter.

Whitening is broken down to three different levels:

1. The dual technique, which couples an in-office procedure with at-home whitening follow-up.
2. The at-home technique alone.
3. Tooth-whitening maintenance alone.

THE DUAL TECHNIQUE: IN-OFFICE WHITENING + AT-HOME WHITENING

In-office whitening uses the most potent amount of hydrogen peroxide, activated even more by high-intensity light wavelengths to bleach deeper and more easily.

This procedure costs anywhere between five hundred and twelve hundred dollars, and it can safely lighten teeth up to ten shades. Unfortunately, that ten-shades-brighter brilliance is usually short-lived. After about three to six months, a majority of the whitening naturally starts to regress. This is why the dual technique works best. The backup of a subsequent at-home technique after the professional treatment puts the active ingredients on the teeth again, so regression is interrupted, thus minimal.

The Evolution of Professional Whitening—From the Laser to the Light Show

In-office whitening has been around since the 1980s. It started with the use of powerful lasers that worked by activating the oxygen in the hydrogen peroxide. Since the laser's power could penetrate well into the dentin, it both sped up the process and gave impressive results.

Unfortunately, along with the whiteness came sensitivity issues. These lasers emitted high amounts of heat—more than 52 degrees Centigrade, which is 122 degrees Fahrenheit—*yeow!* This heat too often caused irreversible changes in teeth, making them permanently sensitive and even occasionally requiring root canals. Despite incremental improvements here and there, the heat continued to cause problems and pain. Even as recently as the late 1990s, newer versions came out that better activated the oxygen (such as the argon CO_2 lasers), but the heat—and the problems associated with it—remained.

In the past few years, lasers have morphed into cooler versions, which are in fact no longer actual lasers but high-intensity white lights, also called arc lamps. They usually use halogen or xenon bulbs that have wavelengths in the 350- to 400-nanometer range. Even though these white lights don't generate anywhere near as much heat as lasers, they still have the power to activate the peroxide's oxygen just as effectively. Look for names like Luma-light (my own choice for in-office) and Zoom. They're used in conjunction with peroxide gels (which the lamp companies usually provide), which are specifically formulated to match—and therefore become activated by—the lights' own particular wavelengths.

The amount of hydrogen peroxide that's used in the gel depends on the individual system a dentist is using. Zoom light usually uses about 25 percent. BriteSmile won't disclose its percentage (but it's known to be less than 25 percent, and the company uses it with its own patented "blue light"). Amounts as high as these have the potential to burn the gum tissues surrounding the teeth. That's why the gums always have to be completely protected and isolated by the professional before any whitening action begins.

Getting the Best Possible Professional Whitening for You

If you decide to have your smile professionally whitened, make sure you choose a reputable aesthetic dentist. As with any kind of treatment, it's vital that you know you're in capable hands. The dentist who filled in your cavities two decades ago and has remained in that era ever since is not the person to go to for state-of-the-art whitening. Try to find a dentist who specializes in aesthetic or cosmetic dentistry. When you meet with her, ask what kind of system she uses. Look for the names that I mentioned, including Zoom and Lumalight. Ask who's going to do the procedure. It should be either the dentist or the hygienist. If it's the hygienist, ask how he was trained and how long he's been performing the procedure. Ask how many patients' teeth he's whitened. If the dentist isn't doing it herself, she should at the very least be overseeing it, checking in on you and your progress every thirty minutes or so.

THE PROFESSIONAL PLAY-BY-PLAY

Ready . . .

The whitening process usually takes about ninety minutes to two hours. Some awkwardness might be involved, but pain should not. If there's pain, it means that your practitioner is doing something wrong, and it probably has to do with gum exposure. The hygienist must cover your gums completely, making sure that everything is sealed off and protected.

A lip retractor gets inserted into your mouth to secure it in its opened position. The good ones allow you to bite down on the back section, which relaxes the jaw muscles. Next, the hygienist will cover the gum tissue with a paint-on rubber dam. The lips and inner cheek area are wiped with a muco-protectant gel. You won't be able to speak (nor should you really move your mouth) for the next few hours, so you should ask for a notepad and a pen with which to communicate. Should an area of the barrier become loosened and cause discomfort, you'll want to alert the hygienist so that the problem can be quickly fixed.

Set . . .

Once the barrier is in place and firmly set, the bleaching can begin. The dentist or trained hygienist will then literally paint the peroxide gel onto each tooth with what looks like a small paintbrush. After all the teeth are coated, the high-intensity light will be aimed directly onto your teeth and left there for about twenty minutes. When the light hits the peroxide, the oxygen within it transforms into free radical oxygen,* making it "superexcited," as I explained earlier. It dives

---

*This is one case where the term *free radical* is a positive one. They're called free radicals because they're molecules with unpaired (as in "free" or "unattached") electrons, just like the free radicals that attack our skin cells. Their tenacity at working their way into the tooth makes them incredibly helpful in stain removal.

into the tooth, penetrates beneath the enamel, and attacks the color pigments. This oxidation procedure causes the pigments to vaporize within the dentin layer, lightening the tooth from within.

Three More Times Around . . .

The white light automatically turns off when the activating time is up. Then the hygienist removes the layer of bleach and brushes on a fresh new coat. Since most professional treatments involve three to four rounds, expect to be open-mouthed, speechless, painted, and lit for about two hours in total. On the off chance that your mouth starts to become sensitive, treatments will be cut down by a round or two.

Go . . .

After a whitening treatment, the teeth remain more porous than usual for at least twenty-four hours. So for the remainder of the day, you shouldn't let yours come into contact with anything that's potentially staining. You'll probably be given something to diminish any sensitivity, but don't be surprised if you experience a few sporadic quick, sharp zings in random spots within your teeth and root. Don't be alarmed (at least no more than feeling the need to cradle your mouth as you would with a toothache). This is just some lingering residue left over from the bleach, and the zings usually dissipate within several hours; they should be gone in the next day or two.

You'll be instructed to abstain from anything that could even remotely cause staining for a good week. This might sound overly cautious, but why leave anything to chance? You just spent close to a month's rent on whitening your smile. If you must drink coffee or any other dark liquid, sip it through a straw. No soy sauce, no tomato sauce, no balsamic vinegar, no cola. No smokes.

WHEN NOT TO WHITEN

- **When you're pregnant:** Research has shown that whitening teeth could possibly harm a fetus.
- **When you're breast-feeding:** There's been no conclusive evidence that's proven whitening to be dangerous when nursing, but there's been no conclusive evidence saying that it's perfectly safe, either. Until we can say for certain that it is harmless for mothers to undergo whitening while nursing, taking such a chance is not advisable.
- **When you're young:** Up until the age of fourteen or fifteen, kids have larger pulps, so whitening is likely to cause sensitivity. Even for patients a few years older who want to whiten, I recommend abbreviated whitening sessions—say, two passes of the procedure instead of the standard four.

Homework

As soon as you see your new whiter teeth, you'll be hit with what I call "the *wow* experience." Your teeth will now have become as many as ten shades whiter, so you won't be able to stop checking them out in the mirror. You'll feel like a new person. It is a great high.

But within a few days, you'll most likely see the whiteness fade somewhat. You can minimize this regression, though, and this is where part two of the dual technique comes into play. Out-of-office whitening (the do-it-yourself follow-up work) means more time with the active ingredients (hydrogen peroxide) on the teeth, and that will subdue regression.

Your dentist might send you home with a tray-and-gel system to use twice a day for three to seven days. Any longer wearing time will cause sensitivity, so its use should be limited—and monitored.

SELF-SERVICE WHITENING: HISTORICAL PERSPECTIVE

The first whitening gels weren't originally created for whitening at all, but for oral care healing. With names like Gly-Oxide and Proxigel, they were formulated to heal mouth sores. But patients were noticing a most pleasing side effect: whiter teeth. So the gels were soon squeezed into bite trays and used instead for their newfound talents. Unfortunately, they did more than whiten; they also caused degradation to the tooth enamel. Their formulas had low pH levels, which encouraged acidic environments in the mouth and caused de-mineralization. This was, of course, a most distressing side effect. So researchers went back into their labs and reformulated the gels, this time with neutral pH levels, and the de-mineralization ceased.

By the late 1980s, dentists offering professionally administered tray-and-gel systems were growing by leaps and bounds. And in 1992, Rembrandt was the first to offer a tray-and-gel system to John and Jane Q. Shopper. Today Rembrandt and other tray-and-gel systems feature boil-and-bite guards and carbamide peroxide gels. Customers are instructed to squeeze the gel into the guard and wear it for an hour and a half.

THERE IS SUCH A THING AS TOO WHITE

Subscribing to the school of too-much-is-never-enough, many people sleep with their trays in their mouths, and experience subsequent sensitivity problems. The truth is, within half an hour, most of the gel is out of the tray and down your throat. Thirty minutes of wear is plenty.

The Verdict on Tray-and-Gels

While tray-and-gels can be very effective on my tougher-stained patients as a three- to four-day in-office procedure follow-up, for the majority of typical staining cases, I do not consider them the most effective treatment. Overuse of the system is a big temptation, and even when used appropriately, sensitivity problems are frequent. Furthermore, there is no one to monitor usage. With all of the advancements in whitening, there are other safer and equally effective options.

Do-It-Yourself Options

Walk into any drugstore, Wal-Mart, Kmart, or Target today and you'll see nearly a dozen at-home whitening products. In May 2001, Crest introduced Whitestrips. About six months after that, Colgate introduced Simply White whitening gel. GoSMILE, which I'd been offering to my patients five years before then, hit the public in spring 2002. In that first year, Americans spent two hundred million dollars on whitening strips. At present, whitening systems and whitening toothpastes are fast approaching the billion-dollar-a-year level. With mass brand products, their levels of actives are safely low (3 percent hydrogen peroxide, versus the professional levels that are above 20 percent). Still, they should be used according to their instructions. If you do so, you should see your teeth brighten by as much as four levels.

CASUAL WHITENING FOR THE COMMITMENT-PHOBE

Let's say your teeth are in fairly decent shape and don't require serious whitening, or even a program of tray-and-gels or strips. Or maybe you've had your teeth whitened but don't want to use an at-home system for fear of potential oversaturation. Still, you wouldn't mind your smile being just a bit brighter. You, then, are the ideal candidate for the portable maintenance whiteners. They're convenient, they're as easy to use as unwrapping a piece of chewing gum (and much better for you), and they take less time to use than it takes to chew that piece of gum.

- **Rembrandt's Whitening Wand:** This product looks and goes on like a lip gloss. Its only drawback is hygiene: Users repeatedly dip and reuse the applicator, allowing bacteria to build up over time.

- **BriteSmile To Go whitening pen:** This looks more like—and even has the consistency of—a click-on brush-tipped lip gloss or concealer. Users click it as many times as needed and apply an ample amount of the gel with the brush tip. Unfortunately, it comes with the same hygiene issues as the Rembrandt Whitening Wand.

- **GoSMILE Daily:** When you pinch this small plastic tube, the hydrogen peroxide formula activates and travels to the sponge-like tip at its end. You brush it over your teeth, wherever you are, for about a minute, then you're done and you can toss it into the garbage.

THIS WHITE'S FOR YOU

Remember, each of us has different tooth colors, depending on our genes and how we've cared for our teeth over the years. It's never too late to make simple changes to brighten our pearly whites, whether it's cutting out or reducing foods that stain, adding foods that fight stains, or introducing an artificial whitening agent. When and if you elect to artificially whiten your teeth, consider cost, convenience, and your desired amount of lightening. Whatever method you choose—always adhere to whatever instructions apply. By taking these steps, you're sure to be smiling more brightly (and more safely) in no time.

WHITENERS AT A GLANCE

	Product	The Experience	Efficacy (1–16 dental shade guide)	Pros	Cons
Strips	Crest Whitestrips	30–45 minutes twice a day, in privacy of your own home, since you can't really wear these in public	4–6	Minimal mess; minimal to moderate sensitivity	Only the six front teeth are covered; not portable; cannot avoid sensitive areas
	Oral-B Rembrandt Whitening Strips	Same as above, except somewhat bulkier	4–6	Same as above	The bulkiness factor
Tray-and-gels	Rembrandt Plus, Rembrandt Dazzling White	Squirt gel into tray, wear at least 30 minutes twice a day, although some suggest overnight	3–4	Keeps gel on teeth for good period of time	Older technology than others; potential soft tissue irritation and tooth sensitivity; unable to target specific areas; often trays don't fit snugly; you'll inevitably swallow some carbamide peroxide, causing mucosal irritation; has the greatest chance of abuse and over-whitening; edges of the teeth can turn gray (translucent)

(continued)

WHITENERS AT A GLANCE (continued)

	Product	The Experience	Efficacy (1–16 dental shade guide)	Pros	Cons
Brush-ons	Colgate Simply White	Like applying Elmer's glue on your teeth; brush off residue when whitening time is completed	1–2	Easy to apply; easy to target specific areas	Nonhygienic—every time you open bottle, bacteria fly in and carbamide peroxide gets out—so best used within 10–14 days
	Crest Night Effects	Apply individually wrapped application with a disposable brush at bedtime, then brush off in morning	4–5	Individual wrapping ensures potency and hygiene; high targetability factor	Feels like you have sweaters on your teeth
	GoSMILE Tooth Whitening on the Go System	Like a toothpick: Unwrap, squeeze, and brush over teeth	4–6	Convenience and hygiene: Toss away after use; high targetability factor; easy to follow regimen; also a breath freshener	More expensive than others
	GoSMILE Advanced B1 Formula	Same as above	Up to 10 in 7 days	Same as above, but also fastest whitening in shortest period of time	More expensive than others

Self-Whiteners, Read This!

Follow Instructions

The outcome of at-home whitening depends on how compliant you are. With these products, your smile can become brighter only if you use them as often as the directions instruct you to. It's not about the intensity, but the frequency of use. We're dealing with a significantly smaller amount of hydrogen peroxide here (6 percent, versus the 20 percent used in dentists' offices), so contact time between the peroxide and your teeth is crucial.

Don't Go Overboard

Instead of weeks, some people make the mistake of whitening for months. Drugstore brands may be milder, but overzealous use of them can cause unattractive, irreversible problems. I cannot stress enough: Do not overbleach. When peroxide is left on the gum area for too long, not only can the area become sore and sensitive, but the gums can even start to recede and separate from the teeth. Not an easy situation to remedy.

Even worse, oversaturation of the peroxide on teeth will eventually begin to vaporize the chromophores, which are the particles that make up a tooth's opacity and color. Once that color fades, the tooth starts to become translucent, and a blue tinge begins appearing along its edges. If it gets to this stage, the tooth's opacity is gone forever. And if that's not enough, oversaturation can also make teeth as brittle and as fragile as eggshells. Once you hit this point, the only remedy is serious dental work, meaning bonding or veneers.

TEN

AESTHETIC IMPROVEMENTS

Nowadays we are able to correct and shape our smiles more easily and with better results than ever before. There are hosts of options that you can explore with your dentist. I have found that constant dialogue with my patients, listening to their concerns and needs, helps ensure satisfaction at the end of the process. It isn't really hand-holding—more like teamwork. The first step is identifying the problem. We do that with a specially designed Aesthetic Evaluation Chart™. Going through it together helps patients get a better grasp on how they feel about their smile and what it is about it that they'd like to change. The next step is to visualize the solution and then choose the most conservative technique to get you there. We visualize the solution using a combination of computer imaging and a diagnostic wax-up; more about these later.

What follows is a rough guide to help you sort through the process of electing and undergoing the most common aesthetic procedures.

IDENTIFYING THE PROBLEM

The details of a new, improved smile are too important to be decided upon by one person who isn't even the owner of the smile in question. As an aesthetic dentist, I have no idea what kind of smile patients want until they tell me. Thus, communication is the name of the game. That's why we go through the process together. The first step is identifying the problem and identifying what the patient would like to change, and which option (or options) are right for that individual.

When telling your dentist what you'd like changed, try to be as specific as possible. Also, provide a complete history of your oral health. Take a moment to jot down any changes your teeth have gone through, whether from braces, previous restorative dentistry, years of wear and tear, or some kind of outside trauma to your teeth. This helps your aesthetic dentist know what you and your smile have been through, and how well you have fared. If you have photos of you at a younger age, before time—or bad dental work—took its toll, bring them in to your dentist. Seeing your original smile can help your dental team return your smile to something more like it used to be. These are the pieces you can contribute to direct your dentist toward giving you the smile you want.

Think about what you want for your future smile relative to one of the three following categories. This will give your aesthetic dentist an understanding of what's beautiful to you and will help direct the restoration in terms of the color, tooth position, and shape.

The Halle Berry smile: Straight, white, and perfect; teeth are uniform in size and shape, perfect edges and symmetrical, tooth color is very white.

The Sarah Jessica Parker smile: Clean, healthy, natural; teeth are clean-looking, not too bright with perfect imperfections (e.g., subtle rotations, offsets, irregular edge).

The Julia Roberts smile: White and natural; this is a combination of the above two descriptions. Here, teeth are a bright white shade with the subtle perfect imperfections.

Once you've provided this information, your dentist should go through a series of analyses that will help you arrive at the best aesthetic option for you.

Facial Analysis

The face drives the shape and position of the teeth. If someone smiles at you and it's a high and wide smile, the teeth might be out of balance or out of proportion to the face. If this is the case, the smile needs to be altered to bring about balance and proportion.

Simply put, the face directs the size of the teeth. And the facial aesthetic drives the tooth size and position. Your dentist will need to look at your face from both the front and the side, the relationship between the lips and the teeth, and the teeth's shape and repositioning.

Head-on Evaluation

By looking at you straight-on, your dentist will evaluate your interpupillary line to your occlusal plane. To translate, this is the horizontal line that runs across the pupils of the eyes. It checks how your eyes line up with the corners of your mouth when you make a full smile.

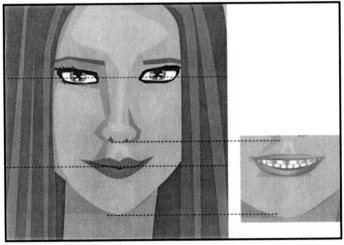

fig. 10.1

Profile Evaluation

The profile is measured with something called Ricketts' E-plane. Ricketts' E-plane is the angle formed when a line is drawn from the tip of the nose to the chin. The "normal" approximation is about ninety degrees. The more obtuse or acute the angle veers, the more pronounced the profile is. If your profile is especially concave, the teeth are usually less visible, which informs the dentist that the teeth should be made bigger. However, if the profile is especially convex, the dentist usually considers making the teeth smaller.

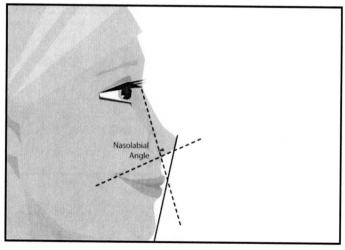

fig. 10.2

Lips and Teeth—Vertical and Horizontal Components

Here's where the dentist investigates your dental composition, examining how your teeth look in relationship to your smile. For instance, when you smile, do you show all the way back to the molars or just past your canines?

When you smile, is it:

- High, showing the whole tooth and some gum?
- Average, showing two-thirds of the tooth?
- Low, showing only the lower edge of the tooth?

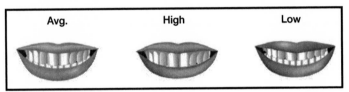

fig. 10.3

Full Smile—Horizontal Component

- How convex or concave is your smile's arch?

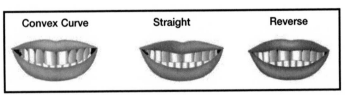

fig. 10.4

- How many teeth can you see when you smile fully—six, eight, ten, or twelve?

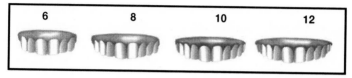

fig. 10.5

- Does your midline skew to the left? To the right? Or is it straight?

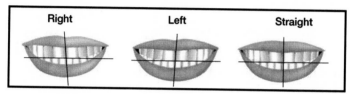

fig. 10.6

- Are your central teeth standing straight? Or do they lean slightly (or not so slightly) to the left or right?

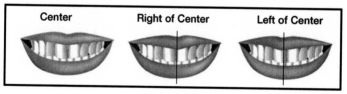

fig. 10.7

- Are there any small open areas near where your teeth and gum meet?
- Phonetic issues: Do you have any type of lisp when you speak? If you do, your tooth alignment could be exacerbating it!

Teeth—Size and Proportion

Lastly, your dentist will take into account your teeth themselves. You may remember that the central incisors are the most dominant followed by the laterals and canines (aka the eyeteeth or bicuspids), on the left and the right.

Proportion of central incisors: The two central upper teeth, the central incisors are the dominant players of the smile. They should be one and a half times the width of the lateral incisors, which flank either side.

Proportion of central to lateral to canine: The three most prominent sets of teeth, the central incisors, laterals, and canines are measured against one another.

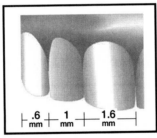

fig. 10.8

Occlusal evaluation: The evaluation of how good your bite is.

Gingival asymmetry: If you have a high smile line, an uneven gum can be more prominent.

VISUALIZE THE SOLUTION

Once you and your dentist have identified the problem or problems, it's time to visualize the solution. In my office, I do this with what's called a diagnostic wax-up. An impression is taken of the mouth and given to a technician, who then perfects the tooth shape and position with a white wax. Spaces get closed up, gum levels are raised (or lowered, or evened out), edges are smoothed, and so on—the ideal smile.

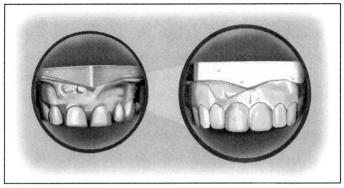

fig. 10.9

Sometimes diagnostic wax-ups can be hard for you, the patient, to fully comprehend, so computer imaging and composite mock-ups can be used to show you what the technician and dentist think your ideal smile could look like. This is when you can weigh in with your opinion, and then adjustments can be made to the replica before anything is done to your actual smile.

TAKE THE TIME TO VISUALIZE

This exploratory part of the process is extremely important: The less you know up front about your options, the greater the chances you'll be talked into more dentistry than is actually necessary. Too often, a dentist will recommend a full face of veneers when all you really need is a combination of techniques, such as whitening and bonding, and a much smaller number of veneers.

A patient came to me after another aesthetic dentist tried to convince her that she needed twenty veneers—ten on top, ten on the bottom—which would have cost her in the neighborhood of forty-five thousand dollars. After reviewing the aesthetic evaluation form together, I asked the woman what bothered her about her smile. She looked at me and said, "First of all, thank you for asking. It's really just the color."

That made it easy to identify the type of smile she wanted: white and natural. (Julia Roberts has the white and natural smile with a beautiful light shade and the perfect imperfections of nature.) Once I saw this woman's diagnostic wax-up, I realized that I only had to make the patient's central incisors more dominant and her canines longer; nothing more. Everything else was in good condition. Rather than twenty veneers, we ended up giving her four—two on her centrals and two on her laterals—with full-mouth whitening and bonding on the canines. The total cost? Less than nine thousand dollars.

AESTHETIC TREATMENT OPTIONS

Porcelain Veneers

Also called porcelain laminates, veneers are undoubtedly the biggest things to hit dentistry since orthodontia. A veneer is a thin layer of porcelain that's personally designed by a specially trained technician to fit over the front and edges of a tooth. Porcelain veneers make it possible for even the most unsightly teeth to be transformed into ideal ones. Their surfaces are so dense that there's virtually no porosity, which makes them impervious to stains and plaque. Though they're quite fragile in the dentist's hands, as soon as they're bonded to the tooth, they become superstrong. Veneers are the technique of choice when you want to add significant length and cover the entire tooth.

The process: First, you and your dentist decide which teeth should be veneered. (Veneers do not come cheap, so when bonding can do the job, such an alternative should be seriously considered.) Next, the surfaces of your selected teeth are reduced (sanded down) by half a millimeter to make room for the ultrathin veneers.

It takes about a week or two for the veneers to be created, so during that time you're fitted with a temporary set, called provisionals, which are made to replicate your smile-to-be. While the veneer technician is busy creating that permanent new smile, you need to be spending this time working your artistic eye and observing the temporary version closely. Look at the color of the teeth, the length of them, the shape of them. This is the time to make sure you like and are comfortable with what you see.

After a few days of the smile dress rehearsal, you return to your aesthetic dentist, who will ask you those same questions: Do you like your tooth color or is it too light—or too dark? Do you like the tooth length? And so on, and so on. If your answer to any of these questions is no, it's important to speak up. Your dentist will then take your concerns back to the technician. Once the final look is approved, impressions of the veneers are taken and are then indexed in the laboratory so that the information can be transferred to the final work.

About a week later, it's time to return for the application of the final veneers. Composite resin cement is used to bond the porcelain to the etched enamel surface. The final step takes place when the laminate is cured to the teeth with a high-intensity light, which takes care of the final hardening (within about sixty seconds). The entire process usually takes two to three hours.

Veneers are right for you if:

- You're changing tooth position and/or tooth size, and they're currently a very difficult color to alter.
- You're really unhappy with the size of your teeth, their positioning, or their dark color.

- Your teeth are noticeably small or thin, and/or noticeably dark.

Advantages of porcelain veneers:

- They're significantly more resistant to staining than bonding. In fact, veneers stain less than natural tooth enamel.
- They're significantly more resistant to chipping than bonding.
- Gum tissues tolerate porcelain well because its surface is so slick and smooth, so there's less likelihood of gum problems arising.
- Veneers are sturdy, and can take the average beating that natural teeth normally endure.

Disadvantages of porcelain veneers:

- A considerable time commitment is required during the application period.
- Veneers are difficult to repair.
- Veneers can be quite costly.
- Veneers irreversibly change the size of your tooth.

Longevity: If properly taken care of, veneers can last twelve to twenty years.

Average cost: Usually around one to two thousand dollars per veneer.

Bonding

Bonding involves the application of a sculptable resin material onto an existing tooth. The composite resin bonding technique is used to both fill in and extend areas, up to a certain point. (More severe cases will require veneers or crowns, which are stronger.) Besides being used to fill cavities, in aesthetic dentistry bonding is used mostly to help reshape teeth, fill in minor gaps, and give teeth better color. Bonding has been practiced for more than twenty years.

The process: First, the surfaces of your teeth are etched with phosphoric acid to create a strong adhesion to the resin. Then the restorative bonding material gets applied. It's a soft and pliable formula, making it easy to brush on. Next, it's cured with a high-intensity light. Once it's hardened, the bonded tooth is then carved and contoured to the ideal tooth form, then finally polished to perfection. If teeth are darkly stained, an opaque whitish layer is also applied and a more durable coat of resin is added to mask the stain completely.

In some cases, such as when a large area is being bonded, the tooth size needs to be reduced to make room for the restorative material that's going to be applied over it. If only a small amount is being added to the tooth or a space is being closed, or, of course, if a tooth is being built *out*, no reduction is necessary.

Bonding is right for you if:

- You want to close small spaces and improve slight rotations (teeth that twist slightly backward or forward).

- You would like to make your teeth moderately longer or wider.
- The color of your teeth is at a level where whitening procedures (both in-office and at-home) aren't strong enough to create a satisfying change.
- You're not a big coffee drinker or smoker—bonding is quite susceptible to staining.

Advantages of bonding: In recent years, bonding has become a relatively quick procedure. Since it usually only entails closing up space and fixing chips and other small imperfections, bonding can be done in one visit. Full-facial bonding has become a rarity since porcelain veneers came onto the scene. (Veneers' durability has made them much more desirable for full-tooth restoration, while bonding is more commonly used to fill in spaces.)

Disadvantages of bonding: If you examine the surface of bonding under a microscope, it looks much like the surface of the moon—very porous. Bonding will pick up all varieties of stains, from lipstick to soy sauce, and aggressive foods such as alcohol can cause peeling and discoloration if you partake often and aren't diligent about brushing afterward.

Longevity: If treated properly and well maintained, bonded teeth can last up to eight years.

Average cost: Bonding usually costs anywhere from five to fifteen hundred dollars per tooth.

Andrea, 39, student

Smile Situation: "My two fifteen-year-old veneers were wearing away, so it was time for new ones. These old veneers were also quite yellow, but at the time, I had no idea just *how* yellow."

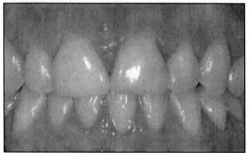

fig. 10.10

Smile Solution: We applied four new veneers, which improved the proportion of her teeth as well as the color. As for the rest, we chose a conservative approach and bonded the canines to close up the spaces. The rest of her teeth were also whitened in order to aesthetically enhance her smile.

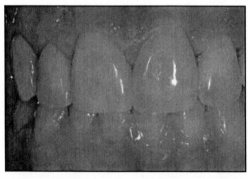

fig. 10.11

Crowns

Crowns are full-coverage reinforcement restorations that bring teeth back to their proper look and function. They're longer lasting, but require more aggressive prep work than a veneer (teeth must be reduced by a 1.5-millimeter reduction as opposed to the 0.5-millimeter reduction required for veneers). Although it's always preferable to preserve the structure of a natural tooth, it isn't always feasible. For example, if an old filling has broken down, once the decay is removed, the tooth's biting surface is undermined, so it needs to be supported by either an onlay, which goes over just the tooth's cusps, or a full-coverage crown.

Crowns can be made up of different materials—porcelain or a combination of porcelain with metal. The type that's chosen not only depends on where the tooth is situated, but what its condition is (how discolored it is and how decayed it is), as well as the condition of the gums. There are three types to choose from:

- **Ceramo-metal:** This is the strongest type of crown. It's usually the most economical, but its disadvantage is that the metal part of it may cast a dark shadow if your gum line recedes. The metal may also affect the color of the porcelain part of the crown.
- **Ceramo-metal crown with porcelain butt joint:** This one can be more costly, but its design better hides the metal, so there's less chance of the metal peeking out eventually.

- **All-porcelain:** An all-porcelain crown looks most like a natural tooth, and there's no metal to be concerned about. That said, it's not as strong as the other two types, so it's slightly more susceptible to chipping. It also costs the most. But, really, at the end of the day, who wants to risk that metal appearing if they don't have to?

The process: First, your tooth or teeth are reduced 1.5 millimeters, as mentioned earlier. An impression is then made of the tooth, from which a life-size model is built from hard stone. A technician then constructs the real crown from the stone model. As with veneers, you're sent home with your provisional set to test. Once the provisional is accepted by both patient and dentist, its important elements are copied into the final crowns.

Each side of the remaining tooth is tapered slightly to hold the crown in place. Next, the crown is tried on to fit comfortably under your gum tissue so any margin between the tooth and crown is hidden. The dentist spends time checking this fit, x-raying to verify it, and adjusting the bite very carefully. It's then finally attached with dental cement or a resin bonding cement.

Crowns are right for you if: Your tooth (or teeth) needs more of a 360-degree type of replacement than one just on its face.

Advantages of crowns:

- Teeth can be whitened or lightened to any desired shade. Very difficult stains can be covered.
- Tooth size or tooth position can be transformed for a better look.

Disadvantages of crowns: Anytime a tooth gets prepared for a crown, there is always the possibility of unnerving it, which means causing severe damage to its nerve. This usually requires a root canal.

Longevity: Crowns have the longest life span of all restorations. They can last fifteen years or more.

Average cost: Twelve hundred to two thousand dollars per tooth.

Alison, 35, pastry chef

Smile Situation: "I hated to smile, my teeth were discolored with spaces. I always put my hand over my face so people couldn't see."

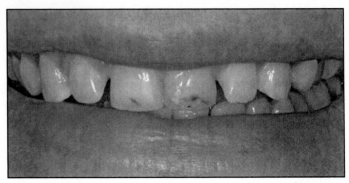

fig. 10.12

Smile Solution: We changed the aesthetics and function of her smile at the same time. Her bite was improved through new crowns, and we put restorations and ceramic jackets on her front teeth.

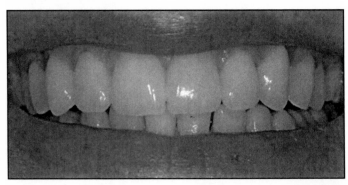

fig. 10.13

David, 53, attorney

Smile Situation: "I'd had two teeth removed from my upper jaw when I was a kid, and that removal affected the entire support system and structure of the rest of my mouth. My teeth met end to end, so they'd been wearing down for thirty years."

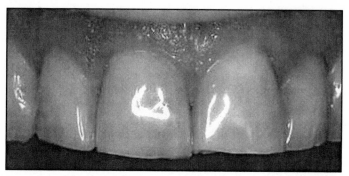

fig. 10.14

Smile Solution: Every tooth in his mouth received a new crown (thirty total), improving the tooth and jaw alignment—which made his smile not only look but also function much better.

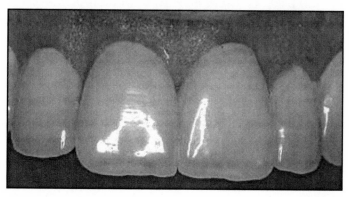

fig. 10.15

Aesthetic Recontouring

Sometimes a tooth simply needs to be shortened or slightly reshaped to bring it back into proportion with the rest of the smile. In these cases, it can be accomplished with a very conservative technique called enamelplasty, which is often used in concert with whitening and/or bonding. As you can probably guess, this downsizing technique is mostly done on central incisors (the "rabbit tooth" effect) and canines when they're too fang-like. The process is fairly simple and straightforward: a handheld piece of fine polishing diamond, in effect, sands the tooth down while polishing the tooth's enamel at the same time. It's not a costly procedure and takes just a few minutes.

Bridges

A bridge is basically a false tooth replacement. In dental-speak, we call it a fixed restoration that replaces a missing tooth. It gets inserted where the missing tooth is supposed to be and is anchored by the teeth on either side of it—hence the name *bridge*.

The process: The bridge is custom-made to fill in the space with a false tooth. The false tooth is then attached by the bridge to the two other teeth on each side of the space.

Next, the teeth are prepared to make room for the new false tooth to accommodate the thickness of the crown's size. The dentist then makes an impression, which serves as the model from which your bridge, false tooth, and crowns then get created by the technician. A temporary bridge is placed in the area to protect teeth and gums while the permanent bridge is being made.

A bridge is right for you if: You want the easiest, most predictable way to fill in a missing tooth's space. When you have a missing tooth, out of the three options (single implant, removable appliance, or fixed bridge), the fixed bridge is still the most viable treatment option, especially when an implant is questionable. However, if you choose a bridge in this case, it will be necessary to crown both teeth on each side of the missing tooth. This trio is called a three-unit bridge.

Advantages of a bridge: A bridge can last for years if done correctly.

Disadvantages of a bridge: Since crowns must be placed on either side of the teeth, it can be a somewhat involved process.

Longevity: It can last for twenty-plus years, depending on how well it's made and the patient's home care.

Average cost: Twelve hundred to two thousand dollars per unit. A three-unit bridge costs anywhere from thirty-six hundred to six thousand dollars.

Implants

Another option for a missing tooth is the single-tooth implant or multiple implants. Implant work is a very exact science usually performed by an oral surgeon or a periodontist, and a prosthodontist or a restorative dentist.

The process: First, the dental team assesses whether you're a good candidate for an implant by examining the quantity and quality of the bone and using X-rays or a dental CAT scan to determine the location and the type of restoration that can go over it. If the location is in your aesthetic zone (toward the front of your mouth) and you have a high smile line, it's important that the implant be positioned perfectly. Placing an implant is a time-consuming surgical procedure. After the original tooth is removed, the area requires a three- to six-month healing period before the implant restoration can go in.

During this healing time, the bone grows in and around the titanium implant, creating a very strong support. However, if the bone or surrounding tissue doesn't grow in as well as hoped, there are grafting procedures that can help with the soft tissue aesthetics.

Implants are right for you if: You're missing one or more teeth and have enough bone in the area to accommodate the anchorage of the implant(s). If you don't have enough bone to do the job, a bone graft might remedy the issue.

Advantages of implants:
- You don't have to alter the adjacent teeth.
- They're easier to maintain. You can floss these restorations because they're individual and not splinted in a bridge.
- Equal distribution of force (it's less taxing on the neighboring teeth).

Disadvantages of implants:
- When it's aesthetically important, it can be difficult to blend in the soft tissue naturally.
- Dental implants can sometimes be rejected, but this happens no more than 2 percent of the time. When it happens, the implant is usually replaced with another one that's slightly larger. Smokers and diabetics have the highest risk of implant failure; with them, the likelihood of failure rises up to 8 to 12 percent.

Longevity: Implants can last fifteen to twenty years.

Average cost: Between the implant placement and the crown, a single tooth implant can cost anywhere from twenty-five hundred to three thousand dollars.

Carrie, 51, emergency room doctor

Smile Situation: "I was never happy with my first set of veneers. Food constantly got stuck in them, which made me nuts!"

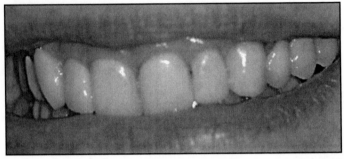

fig. 10.16

Smile Solution: Her high smile line drew attention to her teeth, which needed to be downsized in order to create overall balance in her facial aesthetics. We did this by replacing her old veneers with ones that were better sized and better suited to her face.

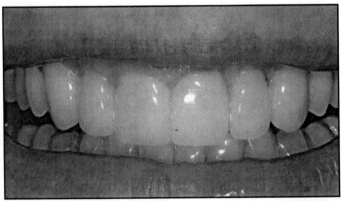

fig. 10.17

Paula, 58, writer

Smile Situation: "I had congenitally missing lateral teeth, which caused large spaces in my smile line. It was time for a change!"

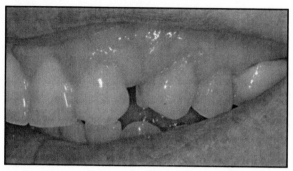

fig. 10.18

Smile Solution: We were able to close the spaces and improve the position and contour by placing ceramic veneers along the upper arch. We placed implants in the areas of the missing teeth, which positioned both arches perfectly. We chose an age-appropriate shade that maintained naturalness.

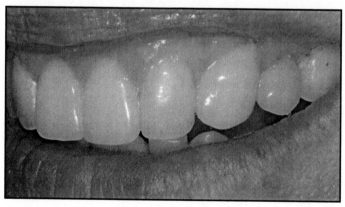

fig. 10.19

Orthodontics

Orthodontics are used when a space needs to be closed or a tooth needs to be moved. Today orthodontics can be practically unnoticeable, since both clear brackets and Invisalign braces are virtually transparent.

The process: To shift teeth into a more desirable arrangement, an orthodontist uses one of two methods: brackets or Invisalign. Brackets involves bonding braces to the front of teeth, which are then connected with wires that direct the teeth toward their goal. Invisaligns, the other option, are clear plastic acrylic shells (which orthodontists call aligners) that snap over the teeth. Invisalign shells are worn in a series, each one slightly different from the one before, for two weeks at a time.

Invisalign is right for you if: Your condition involves tipping or rotation of teeth. Think of it more as a minor type of orthodontics. Also, you need to be an adult with a fully grown jaw. Children can't use this system, because the appliance is prefabricated; everything is manufactured ahead of time, and it's hard to anticipate a child's growth patterns.

Brackets (braces) are right for you if:
- You're below the age of eighteen.
- Your case is more severe. If there are big spaces to close or big movements to make, a fixed appliance (braces) needs to be used.

Advantages of orthodontics: Once the tooth is moved, the need for a restoration (meaning a bonding, veneer, or crown) is less drastic. Orthodontics allow dentists to be more conservative with the restoration, so the need to change a rotation or close a space is minimized.

Disadvantages of orthodontics: Of course, no one likes the idea of wearing something on their teeth, day in and day out. But in just about every case, the ends—straight teeth and great new smile—justify the means.

Longevity: While this period varies greatly according to individual need, the average amount of time orthodontics are worn is about a year. Once the series is done, your orthodontist may give you a positioner, which is a classic retainer, or another aligner similar to the ones you wore during treatment. It's decided on a case-by-case basis.

Average cost: Usually about five to six thousand dollars.

Kathy, 53, finance

Smile Situation: "My nickname in school was The Shark. My teeth weren't bucked or crooked—they went in, and a lot of gum was showing. They were just in bad shape, and they caused me a lot of pain, both psychologically and physically."

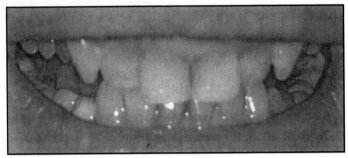

fig. 10.20

Smile Solution: We camouflaged her underlying skeletal problems with orthodontics, periodontics, and prosthodontics—a multidisciplinary approach. This approach included all the areas of treatment that ensured her smile was both functional and beautiful.

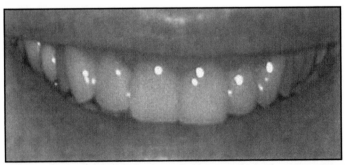

fig. 10.21

WHILE YOU'RE IN THE CHAIR

Here are some things to check when you are undergoing any dental procedure:

- If you're having a crown done, ask for a mirror so you can check to see whether the tooth being worked on looks just like its neighbor. Is it natural looking, and is the gum around it healthy?
- There should be no blackness at the gum line.
- Make sure the dentist takes an X-ray to verify the fit.
- Is the gum area around the restoration area pink and healthy?
- The contact area is the area where the two teeth meet. A perfect contact area is one in which you can floss and clean the restoration perfectly—not too tight, not too loose. A natural contact allows floss to snap right through. But a restoration can alter the contact area, leaving too much space and allowing food to get lodged between the teeth and inflame the gums. Over time, a large space below the contact area can turn into what's called lateral food impaction, which can lead to decay, in addition to gum disease.
- Once the final restoration is in place, all your teeth should touch together with uniform force. It's all about timing and magnitude, the front and back teeth working together harmoniously. For instance, when you slide your jaw forward, your front teeth

(continued)

(While You're in the Chair continued)

touch, but your back teeth don't—this keeps the back teeth from banging into each other. Conversely, when you normally close your mouth and bite down, the back teeth touch slightly harder, so the back teeth are protecting the front teeth from getting worn down. Also, when the bite gets adjusted, a very thin paper (called artist's foil) should be used to help guide the restoration adjustment in all directions of the bite.

- The dentist's office should set you up for a continuous care protocol that includes hygiene appointments, re-calls to check how restorations are doing, and any other work that needs to be taken care of.

SMILE SOLUTIONS: A QUICK REFERENCE GUIDE TO FINDING YOUR FLAW AND FIXING IT

	Problem	Visualize Solution	Appropriate Techniques	Upside	Downside	Cost
Color	Slight yellowness	Whiter smile	In-office whitening, and/or safe, effective over-the-counter whitener	Convenience: in and out in 2–3 hours	Maintenance	$400–800; for at-home product, $40–95
	Very yellow, maybe some brown spots	Whiter smile	Aggressive whitening and spot-bonding	No reducing teeth in size	Chipping, peeling, discoloration	$600–3,000
	Tetracycline staining, gray or dark brown spots	Whiter smile	Porcelain veneers or crowns	Longevity, stain resistance, sturdiness	Costly	$1,500–2,000 per tooth
Tooth Position	Minor gap between centrals	Close gap	Bonding	Easy and fairly quick	Could chip, peel, discolor, pick up stains	$500–1,500
	Wider gaps and teeth that need to be lengthened	Close bigger gap	Orthodontics, bonding, or veneers	Invisalign orthodontics— they're clear!	You'll need a retainer to keep them in new position	Invisalign: $6,000; bonding: $2,000; veneers: $1,200–2,000 per tooth

(continued)

SMILE SOLUTIONS: A QUICK REFERENCE GUIDE . . . (continued)

	PROBLEM	VISUALIZE SOLUTION	APPROPRIATE TECHNIQUES	UPSIDE	DOWNSIDE	COST
Tooth Position (CONTINUED)	Tooth rotated back or forward	Rotated back to harmonize with rest of smile	Orthodontics alone or with veneers and bonding	Orthodontics avoids overcontoured restorations	Need to hold teeth in position long term	See above
Tooth Shape	Minor length problem	Want to make just slightly longer or slight spacing	Bonding	Conservative, no tooth reduction necessary	Could chip	$2,000 per tooth
	Major length problem	Teeth need to be smaller or larger	Veneers	Ceramic surface is stain-resistant and long lasting	Tooth reduction	$1,200–2,000 per tooth
	Substantial size change	Teeth would be properly shaped to face with symmetry at gum level	Periodontal surgery to correct gum level, veneers, and/or bonding	Long-lasting change, dramatic for high-smile patients	More expensive	Surgery: $700–1,500; veneers: $1,200–2,000

ELEVEN

BEAUTY MATTERS

S ure, a great smile can stand alone. But why should it? There are many ways to enhance your smile—giving it the perfect backdrop, so to speak. Here, experts in the beauty field weigh in on the subject.

A MAKEUP ARTIST'S TAKE ON THE SMILE

Celebrity makeup artist Collier Strong, whose clients include Sex and the City's *Kristin Davis, knows firsthand that teeth have a major impact on what your face looks like.*

When I do someone's makeup, I always take not only their skin tone into consideration, but their tooth color as well.

Grayish Teeth

If you had tetracycline as a child or if your teeth just have a genetically gray cast to them, avoid certain reds that have too much blue tones in them, because that really enhances a smile in a negative way. I'm not a big believer in countering the gray with an orange-colored lipstick, though. Instead, choose a cool tone that has a brown base. I call it a warmer cool tone. There are pinks that literally have a brownish hue to them. Think nude pink.

Yellow Teeth

First of all, it's easier to get rid of the yellow than gray, because typically they're stains (versus the tetracycline syndrome), and a good dentist can get rid of them easily. But until you do get them whitened, stick with pink shades that have blue undertones.

The deeper, the darker, or the brighter the lipstick shade you wear, [the more it] is going to make your teeth apparent. If you don't want to draw attention to your teeth, stick with neutral tones, whether it's a balm or lipstick. Even clear lip gloss isn't a great idea. Anything too shiny will draw a lot of attention to your mouth.

Once they're whiter—or if they already are—you can and should wear anything you want, so long as it's appropriate for your skin tone. At this point, it's no longer about what color your teeth are; it's about what color your skin is.

Insider's Tip

Long-wearing lipstick has its moments. It's heaven-sent in certain situations, if it's done well, but if it's not, it's the lipstick from hell that gets on everything. My trick is to use just a bit as a base to stain lips. Blot it on with your finger or a cotton swab, then apply a moisturizing, sheer lipstick in a complementary shade over it. This way, you'll have less incidence of getting it on your teeth or anything else. I don't really pick favorites when it comes to color. I love everything from super-bold red to almost nude. For me, it's more about the effect of the concept I'm creating and less about the lip-color shade.

A SKIN EXPERT'S TAKE ON THE SMILE

World-renowned dermatologist Patricia Wexler has made thousands of women feel better about themselves by bringing a youthful appearance back to their faces. Women whose faces are always in the spotlight trust Pat to keep their complexions smooth, firm, and as line-free as possible.

Cosmetic dermatology and cosmetic dentistry definitely go hand in hand. The nasal labial folds and the chin can recede as we get older, and part of it is due to the recession of the teeth, the gums, and the bone. I always tell my patients that part of the cosmetic unit of the mouth is building the teeth. You have to pay attention to the smile just as you would pay attention to fillers and any other part of the face. Since part of building up the nasal labial fold and the chin is having wonderful teeth, I am a great believer in involving cosmetic dentistry in my patients when we're working on what I call their "plan," in terms of building the laterals, cuspids, and molars, as well as the color of teeth.

A SKIN PROBLEM SOLVER'S TAKE ON THE SMILE

Doris J. Day is an assistant professor of dermatology at New York University and runs a great practice on Manhattan's Upper East Side. When Estée Lauder launched its annex, Beauty Bank, the company called on Day to be its consulting dermatologist for the no-nonsense Good Skin line (she also helped create the products). I asked her to comment on the different skin conditions that can turn up around the smile area.

The smile is the first thing people really notice, because it frames your entire face. I often send patients to a dentist before I do anything in terms of rejuvenation, because if you have good dental work, it can affect your lips and your smile. It can make your lips appear fuller and it can make your mouth more in proportion with your face.

Peri-Oral Dermatitis

Any areas of the face near an orifice have their own specific concerns. Skin around the nose reddens easily, skin around the eyes is really sensitive, and the mouth can experience—and set off—a host of various conditions. Any skin problem around the mouth is called peri-oral dermatitis. It's a broad name for both rashes and acne, and it affects women more than men, probably because women's skin is more sensitive. Also, the chin area is often where women break out when they're premenstrual, so sometimes it's hard to tell what the culprit is.

Redness

If you get redness and pointy bumps around the mouth, it could be hormonal, it could be from your toothpaste, it could be from kissing a man with a beard. There are so many stimuli. The chin area is just very sensitive. If you're very dry there, put a layer of moisturizer ointment like Aquaphor on the area before you brush, then wash off afterward. OTC [over-the-counter] 1 percent hydrocortisone cream will calm down redness, inflammation, and scaling, but use it no longer than about a week, because if used for long periods of time, it can cause thinning. Another thing I recommend for redness: If you use a sulfa-based dandruff shampoo, use a little on the inflamed area of your face; it should calm it down.

Toothpaste Side Effects

There are so many different ingredients in most toothpastes that can cause skin irritation. It could be just about anything—the fragrance, the preservatives—so it's always a good idea to brush your teeth before washing your face, so any possible residue will be washed away.

Dry Lips

Lips don't have oil glands, so they're generally prone to dryness. Along with using lip balm (the less frilly, the better), coat lips with Aquaphor before bed.

Night Drooling

Nighttime drooling can lead to a rash at the corners of the mouth, called perleche. Signs of perleche are usually redness, a bit of scaling, sometimes a fissure (or crack) in skin. Perleche is usually the result of a change in the folds of the mouth, which happens when there's a significant physical change, such as dentures or changes in weight. Weight gain results in a more robust face with a bit of a fold over the chin. And one consequence of significant weight loss is a sunken chin and a deeper fold. Even sun damage can do this, or the shifting of teeth from braces.

However it comes to be, once there's a bit of a crease in that mouth corner, drool can seep through.

And once you have the tiniest fold there, you can accumulate moisture. Just a little fold is enough of a cover to create an environment for yeast to grow and prosper, and you can end up with a condition like a mini diaper rash, usually *Candida*. Derms describe it as "beefy red"; it's an angrier, more intense red than the pinkish red of usual irritation. It's initially treated with an anti-yeast drug with a gentle cortisone cream. Your dentist should be able to help you with that.

TWELVE

NEW FRONTIERS

I magine a toothpaste that can help you fall asleep. Or a mouthwash that helps unclog arteries. A breath spray that prevents the flu. When I look at all the technological discoveries popping up in the oral care industry, I truly believe we're only starting to scratch the surface of the smile beauty world. As this category continues to be explored, you won't believe some of the technologies that are coming down the pike. And you certainly won't want to miss out on them.

SMILECEUTICALS

How many times have you heard the phrase, *It kills the germs that cause bad breath*? Most standard mouthwashes, as well as toothpastes and other oral care products you see on the shelves today, market their powers of killing cavity-causing or bad-breath bacteria. But

197

there's a big problem with this way of thinking. Any oral product or treatment aimed at killing bacteria actually fractures the health of the oral environment. We *need* those "bad" bacteria. They're part of the natural balance of our mouths.

Instead of attacking bacteria, products need to promote a balanced environment within the mouth. This can be accomplished by introducing more vitamins and other nutrients via oral care product formulations. By doing this, the inside of your mouth develops a stronger natural immune response, making it less vulnerable to bacteria.

This is the future of oral care, and I call it smileceuticals. Just like the nutriceuticals in the food market and the cosmeceuticals on the skin care shelves, smileceuticals are what you get when you combine oral care and overall wellness. Our mouths are a great place to receive vitamins and anti-oxidants that benefit the immune system of our entire bodies. The same way that our small intestines have strong uptake properties with which to absorb these vitamins, so does our oral mucosa (the mouth's mucous membrane).

Smileceuticals use a combination of natural ingredients that, together, promote a healthy bacterial balance inside the mouth. While the old-school approach to oral care is to use chemicals that in effect kill, we now know how to implement natural ingredients that promote a healthy balance of good and bad bacteria. Smileceuticals' natural blend of biologically active ingredients create a synergy of anti-oxidant, anti-inflammatory, anti-bacterial, and immune response enhancement with healing and repair qualities.

One of the agents that promotes exactly the kind of healthy bacterial balance I'm talking about is probiotics, a word you're going to see more and more, and not just in the oral care arena.

Imagine if a toothpaste or rinse could reinfuse the mouth with beneficial bacteria, enabling the existing bacteria to better metabolize sugars and hold their own against negative ones, such as *Streptococcus mutans* (the bacteria that create the acid that, in turn, causes decay). Every time you brushed or gargled, you'd be putting back in your mouth more of the bacteria that need to be there. Instead of killing bacteria, you would be leveling the environment. This would be a probiotic toothpaste.

As with revolutionary anti-oxidants and chewing gum that promote stronger gum tissue, Europe and Asia are already using probiotics.

Mike Pellico runs Laclede laboratories, the company that makes Biotène toothpastes and rinses—products that target dry mouth. Instead of using chemicals to oxygenate the saliva, Biotène uses natural enzymes to inhibit the growth of bacteria, so the mouth can create more saliva on its own.

A major proponent of probiotics, Pellico says, "Everything's anti-microbial these days: soaps, anti-microbial hand creams, anti-microbial toothpastes. It's like a horse race—'We kill more bacteria than you do!'—but we now know that bacteria's our first line of defense against opportunistic infections, like yeast infections. We need to switch from anti-microbial to probiotic. Let's stop talking about killing; let's talk about making things healthy again, because a healthy mouth is not a sterile mouth. A healthy mouth is one where the body has the right mix of bacteria in it, because that's your first line of defense."

SUPER-DUPER ANTI-OXIDANTS

You've probably heard of free radicals, the hazardous environmental elements—the sun, smoke, or pollution—that attack skin cells and cause premature aging. Free radicals are found in the bacteria that cause everything from damage to the cell membrane to, ultimately, oral cancers. Anti-oxidants have been used for years to defend every vital organ, including skin, against free radical damage, and they've also long been known for their ability to defend against dental issues such as gum disease and periodontal disease. Additionally, anti-oxidants have powerful healing and reparative influence on the soft tissues of the oral cavity (the tongue, the gums, the inner lining of the cheeks), along with an increase in overall well-being.

The known anti-oxidants are the vitamins A, C, E, and K, among others. In oral care, these vitamins help reduce plaque, prevent gum disease, aid in wound healing, and promote collagen synthesis. In the past few years, however, new breeds of anti-oxidants have started appearing in supplements and formulas whose powers exceed the others by leaps and bounds.

Coenzyme Q10

You might have heard of this one already. CoQ10 has been lauded for its powers in increasing the body's resistance to disease. In cardiologist Stephen T. Sinatra's book *The Coenzyme Q10 Phenomenon,* he writes, "It is my belief that the Coenzyme Q10 not only improves the quality of life with patients with diseases, but also saves lives." While many take it as a nutrient to fight aging, CoQ10 is also used for a wide variety of serious degenerative diseases, such as heart disease, high blood pressure, cancer, diabetes, and periodontal disease. Basically, its magic lies in its powers to support any tissue in the human body in need of repair or assistance.

Pycnogenol

The Europeans are decades ahead of us in researching the powers of this new class of anti-oxidants, and one of the most powerful products they have developed is Pycnogenol. Extracted from the bark of the maritime pine tree that grows along the coastline of southern France, its powers were first discovered hundreds of years ago as a cure for scurvy.

Fast-forward to the 1970s, when a Switzerland-based company, Horphag Research, took the bark from this tree that's grown pesticide-free, fertilizer-free, and pollutant-free, and extracted Pycnogenol from it. This stuff has been proven to protect against free radicals about twenty times more powerfully than vitamins C, E, A, CoQ10, and grape seed. Pycnogenol has helped in alleviating the broadest set of disparate conditions, from diabetes to blood clotting to, yes, gum disease.

Pycnogenol promotes overall wellness and overall health in the mouth. It's been proven to seal capillaries and bind collagen to decrease inflammation in the mouth, reduce plaque accumulation on teeth, and improve overall circulation.

Revolutionary mouthwashes and oral sprays containing both CoQ10 and Pycnogenol are about to hit the market. These cutting-edge products will keep gums and teeth healthy and stronger, keep breath fresher, and even help reduce the incidence of cavities.

Using these products will be like taking a multivitamin, but one that tastes great and has fantastic oral benefits. In the not-too-distant future, there will be toothpastes, sprays, and rinses packed with anti-oxidants that will keep gums healthy, remove free radicals from inside the mouth, and improve overall health. Using these will bring about a stronger immune environment inside the mouth and throughout the entire body.

DEFYING CAVITIES

Forty billion cavities are filled each year in the United States. That makes up 50 percent of the dental industry and 5 percent of overall health care. But if dentistry continues to advance at the rate it is these days, cavities could be a thing of the past before we hit the next decade.

Out of all the strains of bacteria living in our mouths (which number from three to five hundred), only one, *Streptococcus mutans,* is responsible for tooth decay. This bacterium converts sugar into enamel-corroding lactic acid, which is what causes a cavity in a tooth. A Florida-based company called Oragen has developed a genetically modified strain of the bug that doesn't make lactic acid, so, in effect, *look, Ma, no cavities.*

"We all have *Strep mutans* in our mouths from the age of two or three," explains Oragen's founder Jeffrey Hillman, DMD, PhD. "Our strain would simply kick out the disease-causing strain and take over the niche on the tooth surface of *Strep mutans.*"

The way it works is remarkably simple: Your dentist sprays a rinse that contains the strain (whose code name is BCS3-L1) after a cleaning. And all you need to do to activate it is eat something with sugar in it.

The idea of using good bacteria to fight bad bacteria is nothing new—Louis Pasteur came up with it more than a hundred years ago. And while nature could provide similar bacterial replacements, no one's ever been lucky enough to find a perfect one, explains Hillman. "The difference between what people have done in the past with replacement therapy and what we've done is that we've taken advantage of new tools in DNA technology that have become available over the last fifteen years or so and tailored our strain so that all the properties that you would *want* are in the strain."

So far, this new treatment has only been tested on laboratory rats, but after a year, the rats, who feasted on sugar-intensive diets, remained acid- and cavity-free. Human testing has recently begun, and if it's green lights all the way—something Hillman is very optimistic about—cavities will be squirted instead of drilled, at a cost comparable to a filling or a crown.

But don't toss your floss just yet. "All we're doing is changing the *Strep mutans*," emphasizes Hillman. "The other 299 or 499 strains are going to be the exact same as they were before, which include the ones that cause periodontal disease. So if you have bacteria that causes periodontal disease, if you don't brush and floss, you're still going make yourself prone to that."

INSIDER INFO

One of the newest strengtheners for tooth re-mineralization is a compound made up of calcium, phosphorus, silica, and sodium that has strengthened millions of bone fractures. Taking the knowledge that bones and teeth are of similar makeup (and therefore might be strengthened similarly) led to the creation of NovaMin. When NovaMin comes into contact with water or saliva, it instantly releases billions of mineral ions that aid in the natural tooth re-mineralization process. We're currently working on a desensitizing toothpaste that will contain Novamin.

THE FUTURE OF WHITENING

Today one hundred million Americans are whitening their teeth. And whether they are professional applications or over-the-counter products, all whitening agents have room for improvement. Future advancements will help people whiten their teeth faster, for longer, with fewer side effects.

Self-Whitening Improvements

While in-office whitening plus at-home maintenance continues to be the best way to get teeth whiter, there are ongoing advancements in the at-home category. Be on the lookout for:

- **Whitening maintenance:** Whitening systems are too strong to use for maintenance on a daily level. Instead, we need something that prevents regression and stains—but in a very safe, gentle way with low actives. Such whitening maintenance products—which are gentle enough to use every day without the risk of destroying the dentin—are already available among the GoSMILE line, but more available options will be hitting drugstore shelves soon.
- **Whiter, brighter—for longer:** As I discussed earlier, paint-on whiteners are the safest of all whiteners, and with better polymer gel resin technology, the

hydrogen peroxide will stay on teeth longer. Also on the way is a time-released gel that contains 6 percent hydrogen peroxide when applied, but increases to 10 percent over the course of five to ten minutes—cutting the time you have to keep the agent on your teeth significantly.

- **Multitasking:** Why only whiten when you can get stronger teeth, too? Technicians are experimenting with using calcium phosphates in whitening gels that would help keep teeth healthy. And this kind of benefit wouldn't be just for those whose teeth had become brittle from too much whitening gel; it would benefit anyone whose teeth could use some hardening, which is, well, everyone.

- **Improved targetability:** Ideal whitening strips would target the area you want to whiten and not the areas you don't, such as sensitive gums. Soon strips will have scalloped edges to follow along gum lines, and they'll be tailored to fit your specific gum line pattern.

- **Post-whitening toothpaste:** Given the whitening explosion, who wouldn't appreciate a toothpaste that could help with any side effects that may have arisen through whitening, such as the softening of the tooth enamel or sensitivity? Necessary actives, like fluoride and potassium nitrate, can be found in Sensodyne toothpaste with fluoride and my pending GoSMILE professional toothpaste.

Better Care in the Chair

In-office whitening is a very impressive procedure, but some improvements can still be made. Here's what the experts are working on:

- **Less time in the chair:** Now it's about ninety minutes. Eventually, it'll be as quick as half an hour.
- **Higher concentration of the actives:** Of course, they'll remain safe and gentle, but the higher concentration will bring about both faster and brighter whitening.
- **Less sensitivity:** While a professional whitening treatment doesn't necessarily hurt, it can cause some pretty uncomfortable sensitivities. We're trying to make that possibility not even a possibility.
- **Less expense:** Just like the case of computers, as technology improves, the price will go down.
- **Less regression:** As technology improves, regression should also occur less.
- **Improved follow-up maintenance:** Follow-up products are being launched that are easy to use and fit people's lifestyles. More such innovations are on the way.

Today more importance than ever is being attached to achieving a great smile. The future of smile beauty—and that certainly includes oral care—is bright, and thanks to innovative research and technology in this field, it is becoming easier and easier to maintain the health and integrity of your greatest asset—your smile!

GREAT MOMENTS IN DENTAL HISTORY: A TIME LINE

Stick and Stone Age: Humans find ways to clean their
teeth with twigs and sticks that are mashed at one end,
creating a spread-out, flatter surface with which to brush
what few teeth they have.

1498—Toothbrush origins: The first toothbrush is created in
China when hog bristles are embedded into a bone handle.
In true Marco Polo fashion, once it hits the Continent, Euro-
peans run with the idea and make it their own, just like pasta.

1540s—Sugar invades England: When sugar starts to be
imported to Europe and purified into white crystalline,
one of its most famous victims is Queen Elizabeth I, who
ends up with a mouthful of black teeth as a result.

1700s—Tooth donors: Not that the success record was very high, but in the eighteenth century, a lost tooth was sometimes replaced by an extracted tooth from another person. This just reeks of an unfair, archaic class system.

1774—False teeth created: Two Frenchmen, a pharmacist and a dentist, design the first set of porcelain teeth. Subsequently, in 1808, an Italian dentist invents a single porcelain tooth that's embedded with a platinum pin.

1790—The advent of the dental chair: Boston-based Josiah Flagg designs the first dental chair, by nailing an adjustable headrest to the back and making one armrest large enough to hold a few dental instruments.

1799—George Washington's other lie: By the time he takes office, the Father of Our Country has lost nearly all his teeth. Four sets of false teeth are made for him, but none is made of wood. (How *could* it be? Think of wood when it gets wet.) His dentist made them from gold, hippopotamus tusk, and elephant ivory with a few actual human teeth thrown in for good measure. The sets prove to be too short, though. When he poses for what will undoubtedly be his most famous portrait, the Father of Our Country's mouth is so sunken that gobs of cotton need to be stuffed into his mouth to fill it out.

1815—First floss: While traces of dental floss have been found in teeth of prehistoric humans, Levi Spear Parmly, a New Orleans dentist, gets the star for creating the first modern dental floss using silk thread.

1824—First toothpaste additives: Dentists start fiddling around with ways to make toothpaste more user-friendly. Soap is first added in 1824. A few decades later, chalk is mixed in. In 1873, Colgate adds a pleasant flavoring and puts it in jars. In 1892, a Connecticut dentist is the first to put it in a tube, calling it Dr. Sheffield's Creme Dentifrice. A few years later, Colgate gets into the tube business and names its product Colgate Dental Cream.

1840s—Mouth peace: Horace Wells introduces the use of nitrous oxide for dental anesthesia. About sixty years later, the first anesthesia machines start appearing in dental practices.

1866—First lady: Lucy Beaman Hobbs becomes the first woman to receive a dental degree, from the Ohio School of Dentistry.

1880—First electric toothbrush: A dentist named Dr. Scott markets the first electric toothbrush, advertising it as "permanently charged with electro-magnetic current." The first truly effective one is developed in Switzerland just after World War II, but it's not until the 1960s that Squibb and General Electric are able to successfully market electric toothbrushes in the United States.

1905—Feeling nothing: After decades of using cocaine as an anesthetic, Alfred Einhorn, a German chemist, synthesizes a substitute, naming it novocaine.

1945—The flow of fluoride: The notion of adding fluoride to city water supplies becomes a reality when two cities—Newburgh, New York, and Grand Rapids, Michigan—introduce sodium fluoride into their public water systems. At the same time, a group of Wisconsin-based dentists succeed at getting the entire state's water system fluoridated. After substantial testing shows that fluoride reduces incidence of cavities by as much as two-thirds, the U.S. Public Health Service in 1951 urges the entire country to fluoridate public drinking water.

1955—Creamy filling: Michael Buonocore invents white composite fillings at the Eastman Dental Center in Rochester, New York.

1967—Savings bonds: Dr. Buonocore starts off the bonding revolution by discovering how to bond to the tooth's surface by the acid-etch technique. Until now, a very thin layer of porcelain would simply be cemented to a tooth, so it didn't stay on for very long. The acid-etch technique changes that forever.

1970s—The most infamous dental record: Among all of the evidence gathered for serial killer Ted Bundy's murder trials, the bite marks he leaves on the buttocks of victim Lisa Levy play prominently in the case. To keep this nefarious mastermind from, in effect, grinding his own evidence away, the authorities obtain a search warrant that enables them to surprise Bundy and force a dental impression out of him. When a transparent sheet with an enlarged photo of Bundy's teeth is placed over the victim's bite mark, there appears to be no doubt that he left his mark on his victim.

1981—Public bonding: NYU dentist Harold Horn works with ceramist Adrian Jurim to create the porcelain veneer technique. Bonding soon goes mainstream, and the revolution begins.

1985—Firmly planted: A Swedish inventor named Branemark creates dental implants.

1987—Self-help: Harold Heymann publishes the first paper documenting the beneficial results of an at-home whitening system using a bite tray and gel.

1990s—National awareness: The side-by-side discoveries of porcelain veneers and professional whitening prompt a nationwide increase in dental visits as people with imperfect smiles discover how easy it is to improve theirs. Superwhite Chicklet teeth become the smile of choice.

1995—Laser show: Lasers are introduced as a powerful way to activate hydrogen peroxide for professional in-office whitening procedures. Meanwhile, at-home whitening systems are given to patients by their dentists, both to maintain a professional job and to bump an already bright smile up a notch or two. Within five years, the at-home whitening industry will have become a four-hundred-million-dollar one.

2000—New lighting: High-intensity white lights begin to replace the laser for in-office whitening. And speaking of replacements, the Hollywood full-wattage smile starts to become passé as a shift in desire to a more natural-looking set occurs.

2001—Invisalign debuts: This new invisible orthodontic technology removes the ugly stigma that has always been attached to braces.

2001—Strip ease: Crest launches Whitestrips, with Colgate fast on its heels. These two launches elevate the concept of teeth whitening to the mass level for the first time.

2002—Portable whitening: GoSMILE's patented ampoule systems launches at retail. The system was available to Dr. Levine's patients from 1996.

2003—Über-ceramics: With the advent of stronger ceramics, dentists finally can offer restorations that are not only more aesthetically pleasing but also strong.

GLOSSARY

Acidifying: Anything with a pH level lower than neutral, which should be ingested at measured levels when it comes to food.

Aesthetic zone: The front part of the smile that's most visible, so aesthetics matter more (versus farther back in the smile).

Alkalinizing: Something with a pH level higher than neutral, which is a positive thing when it comes to food.

Amalgam: The industry word for "filling," meaning it's an amalgamation of different metals (tin, silver, copper).

Anaerobic bacteria: Bacteria that live in areas without oxygen and thus promote bad breath and gum disease.

Arc lamp: The high-intensity lamp that activates hydrogen peroxide during an in-office whitening procedure without heat.

Autoclave: A heat sterilizer in the dentist's office.

Barrier control: The plastic wrapping over all dental supplies to keep them protected before use.

Bonding: A type of restorative dentistry in which fronts and edges of teeth can be whitened, elongated, and widened to a certain extent.

Bridge: A splinted unit that replaces a tooth and is supported by a natural tooth (abutment) on either side.

Cariogenic: Something that promotes cavities.

Contact area: The area where teeth that are next to each other meet.

Crown: A full-coverage restoration that supports the tooth 360 degrees. It can be made from ceramic, metal, or a combination of the two.

Dentin: Beneath the enamel, where a tooth's color and opacity comes from.

Enamel: A tooth's rock-hard, clear protecting surface.

Endodontic lesion: When a nerve dies in a tooth, causing biting to be painful and swelling, requiring a root canal.

Endodontist: A root canal specialist.

Flap surgery: The surgical procedure that's performed when scaling and root planing aren't enough to eliminate pockets.

Gingival symmetry: An even gum line.

Gingivitis: A milder form of periodontal disease. Also called gum disease.

Hydrogen peroxide: The bleaching agent used in all tooth whitening, which is stabilized either by a carrier such as carbamide peroxide, or by a delivery system such as the one in GoSMILE ampoules.

Implant: A type of restorative dentistry that involves replacing a missing tooth (or teeth) but that's anchored in below the gum line through the jaw.

Inlays and onlays: Indirect restoratives that are used when decay in a tooth requires more than a filling or amalgam but not enough to require a crown.

Irreversible pulpitis: An inflamed nerve that's past the point of rescue and heading down the road to root canal city.

Malocclusion: An uneven bite.

Mandible: The lower jaw of teeth.

Maxilla: The upper jaw of teeth.

MPD: Myofascial pain dysfunction, which is muscle soreness due to a bite problem.

Orthodontics: Tooth movement through applied force that either tips or bodily moves a tooth in the desired direction.

Osteoclastic activity: The loss of bone.

Oversaturation: When a whitening product's active ingredient penetrates a tooth's enamel for an overextended period of time, resulting in unsupported tooth enamel, erasing its dentin's pigment and structure.

Oxidizing: Reduction reaction through the power of oxygen and an unpaired electron.

Oxygenating: The action of bringing oxygen into an area, such as the mouth.

Periodontitis: Bone loss associated with gum inflammation.

Plaque: Bacteria film formed with a glyco-protein base (especially sugars and carbohydrates) left on unbrushed and unflossed teeth that turns sticky and hardens.

Pocket: What the small crevices can grow into when they become enlarged to more than five millimeters deep and bleed upon probing.

Porcelain veneers: A thin laminate or layer of porcelain bonded onto the natural tooth surface to change tooth position, tooth color, and tooth shape.

Pulp: Provides nutrients and blood supply to the innermost area of the tooth.

Reversible pulpitis: An inflamed nerve that can return to health.

Root planing: Removing plaque (bacterial endotoxin) from beneath the gum line.

Scaling: Removing tartar (hardened plaque) from above the gum line.

Sulcus: The small crevice between the teeth and the gums.

Tartar: Hardened plaque above the gum.

Tray-and-gel whitening system: The first type of whitening system that could be used at home.

TMJ disorder: Temporomandibular joint disorder, which refers to an internal problem in the joint in addition to the muscle.

Volatile sulfur compounds: Aka VSCs; the compounds in your mouth that cause bad breath.

Whitening ampoule: An at-home or on-the-go whitening delivery system in which hydrogen peroxide stays inertly potent until activated at time of use.

Whitening strip: An at-home whitening system where the active ingredient is delivered in a gel-like form via a tape-like strip.

RESOURCE GUIDE

*The following organizations can provide authoritative
information on many different areas of dentistry:*

Academy of General Dentistry (AGD)
211 East Chicago Avenue, Suite 900
Chicago, IL 60611-1999
Phone: (888) AGD-DENT (888-243-3368)
Fax: (312) 440-0559
www.agd.org

*A resource for practitioners and for consumers looking for
reliable dental health information.*

American Academy of Esthetic Dentistry (AAED)

401 North Michigan Avenue

Chicago, IL 60611

Phone: (312) 321-5121

Fax: (312) 673-6952

E-mail: aaed@smithbucklin.com

www.estheticacademy.org

A membership organization dedicated to raising awareness about and upholding the standards of dental aesthetics as related to overall oral health care.

American Academy of Implant Dentistry (AAID)

AAID Headquarters Office

211 East Chicago Avenue, Suite 750

Chicago, IL 60611

www.aaid-implant.cnchost.com

A membership organization dedicated to advancing the art and science of implant dentistry. It provides information to the public and practitioners, provides educational opportunities, and serves as the credentialing standard for implant dentistry.

American Academy of Pediatric Dentistry (AAPD)

211 East Chicago Avenue, Suite 700

Chicago, IL 60611-2663

Phone: (312) 337-2169

Fax: (312) 337-6329

www.aapd.org

A membership organization representing the specialty of pediatric dentistry.

American Academy of Periodontology (AAP)

737 North Michigan Avenue, Suite 800

Chicago, IL 60611-2690

Phone: (312) 787-5518

Fax: (312) 787-3670

www.perio.org

A member association of dental professionals specializing in the prevention, diagnosis, and treatment of diseases affecting the gums and supporting structures of the teeth and in the placement and maintenance of dental implants.

American College of Prosthodontists (ACP)

211 East Chicago Avenue, Suite 1000

Chicago, IL 60611

Phone: (312) 573-1260

Fax: (312) 573-1257

www.prosthodontics.org

The official sponsoring organization for the specialty of prosthodontics.

American Dental Association (ADA)

211 East Chicago Avenue

Chicago, IL 60611-2678

Phone: (312) 440-2500

www.ada.org

A professional association of dentists committed to the public's oral health, ethics, and science, and to the professional advancement of practitioners.

GoSMILE
110 East 42nd Street, Suite 1301
New York, NY 10017
(877) 8-SMILES
www.gosmile.com

Dr. Levine's patented home whitening system. Its Web site features GoSMILE whitening products, as well as the science behind them, guidelines on their proper use, articles, and testimonials.

The following list is a compilation of the best dental schools in the country. These institutions can help direct you to the high quality dental care in your area:

University of Alabama
1919 7th Avenue South, Room 406
Birmingham, AL 35294
(205) 934-4720
www.dental.uab.edu

Arizona School of Dentistry & Oral Health
5850 East Still Circle
Mesa, AZ 85206
(480) 219-6000
asdoh.atsu.edu

University of Arkansas—Fort Smith
5210 Grand Avenue
P.O. Box 3649
Fort Smith, AR 72913
(479) 788-7000
www.uafortsmith.edu

University of Arkansas—Little Rock
4301 West Markham
Mail Slot 619
Little Rock, AR 72205
(501) 686-5730
www.uams.edu

UCLA School of Dentistry
10833 Le Conte Avenue
Los Angeles, CA 90095
(310) 825-2337
www.ucla.edu

University of California—San Francisco School of Dentistry
513 Parnassus Avenue, S630
San Francisco, CA 94143
(415) 476-1323
dentistry.ucsf.edu

University of the Pacific Arthur A. Dugoni School of Dentistry
2155 Webster Street
San Francisco, CA 94115
(415) 929-6400
www.dental.pacific.edu

University of Southern California School of Dentistry
925 West 34th Street
Los Angeles, CA 90089
(213) 740-2800
www.usc.edu

University of Colorado School of Dentistry
4200 East 9th Avenue, Box C-284
Denver, CO 80262
(303) 315-8752
www.uchsc.edu

University of Connecticut School of Dental Medicine
263 Farmington Avenue
Farmington, CT 06030
(860) 679-2325
sdm.uchc.edu

Nova Southeastern University College of Dental Medicine
3200 South University Drive
Fort Lauderdale, FL 33328
(800) 541-6682
dental.nova.edu

University of Florida College of Dentistry
P.O. Box 100405
Gainesville, FL 32610
(352) 392-2911
www.dental.ufl.edu

Medical College of Georgia School of Dentistry
1120 15th Street
Augusta, GA 30912
(706) 721-0502
www.mcg.edu

University of Hawaii—Manoa, Dental Hygiene
2500 Campus Road
Honolulu, HI 96822
(808) 956-8111
www.hawaii.edu

Idaho State University, Dental Hygiene
Campus Box 8048
Pocatello, ID 83209
(208) 282-3796
www.isu.edu

University of Illinois—Chicago College of Dentistry
801 South Paulina Street
Chicago, IL 60612
dentistry.uic.edu

Indiana University School of Dentistry
1121 West Michigan Street
Indianapolis, IN 46202
(317) 274-7957
www.iusd.iupui.edu

University of Iowa College of Dentistry
Iowa City, IA 52242
(319) 335-9650
www.dentistry.uiowa.edu

Johnson County Community College, Dental Hygiene
12345 College Boulevard
Overland Park, KS 66210
(913) 469-8500
www.jccc.edu

Wichita State University, Dental Hygiene
1845 North Fairmount
Wichita, KS 67260
(316) 978-3614
www.wichita.edu

University of Louisville School of Dentistry
501 South Preston
Louisville, KY 40202
(502) 852-5096
dental.louisville.edu

Louisiana State University School of Dentistry
1100 Florida Avenue, Box 141
New Orleans, LA 70119
(504) 619-8500
lsusd.lsuhsc.edu

**University of Louisiana—Monroe Department of
Dental Hygiene**
700 University Avenue
Monroe, LA 71209
(318) 342-1621
www.ulm.edu

University of Maine—Augusta, Dental Health Programs
46 University Drive
Augusta, ME 04330-9410
(207) 621-3000
www.uma.edu

University of New England, Dental Hygiene
Westbrook College Campus
716 Stevens Avenue
Portland, ME 04103
(207) 797-7261
www.une.edu

University of Maryland—Baltimore College of Dental Surgery
666 West Baltimore Street
Baltimore, MD 21201
www.dental.umaryland.edu

Boston University Goldman School of Dental Medicine
One Sherborn Street
Boston, MA 02215
(617) 353-2000
www.dentalschool.bu.edu

Harvard School of Dental Medicine
188 Longwood Avenue
Boston, MA 02115
(617) 540-5044
www.hsdm.harvard.edu

Tufts University School of Dental Medicine
One Kneeland Street
Boston, MA 02111
(617) 636-6828
www.tufts.edu/dental

University of Detroit Mercy School of Dentistry
8200 West Outer Drive
Detroit, MI 48219-0900
(313) 993-1000
www.udmercy.edu

University of Michigan School of Dentistry
1011 North University
Ann Arbor, MI 48109
(734) 763-6933
www.dent.umich.edu

University of Minnesota School of Dentistry
515 Delaware Street SE
Minneapolis, MN 55455
(612) 624-8400
www.dentistry.umn.edu

**University of Mississippi Medical Center School of
Dentistry**
2500 North State Street
Jackson, MS 39216
(601) 984-6000
dentistry.umc.edu

University of Missouri—Kansas City, School of Dentistry
650 East 25th Street
Kansas City, MO 64108
(816) 235-2100
www.umkc.edu/dentistry

Montana State University—Great Falls College of Technology, Dental Hygiene
2100 16th Avenue South
Great Falls, MT 59405
(800) 446-2698
www.msugf.edu

Creighton University School of Dentistry
2802 Webster Street
Omaha, NE 68178
(402) 280-5060
www.creighton.edu

University of Nebraska Medical Center College of Dentistry
40th and Holdrege Street
P.O. Box 830740
Lincoln, NE 68583
(402) 472-1301
www.unmc.edu

University of Nevada—Las Vegas, School of Dental Medicine
1001 Shadow Lane Campus
MS 7410
Las Vegas, NV 89106
(702) 774-2520
www.unlv.edu/dentalschool

New Hampshire Technical Institute, Dental Hygiene
31 College Drive
Concord, NH 03301
(603) 271-6484
www.nhti.edu

University of Medicine and Dentistry of New Jersey,
New Jersey Dental School
110 Bergen Street, P.O. Box 1709
Newark, NJ 07101
(973) 972-7539
www.dentalschool.umdnj.edu

San Juan College, Dental Hygiene
4601 College Boulevard
Farmington, NM 87402
(505) 326-3311
www.sanjuancollege.edu

University of New Mexico, Dental Hygiene
2320 Tucker, NE
Albuquerque, NM 87131
(505) 272-4513
www.unm.edu

Columbia University Medical Center School of Dental
and Oral Surgery
630 West 168th Street
New York, NY 10032
(212) 305-3478
www.columbia.edu

New York State University—Buffalo School of Dental Medicine
315 Squire Hall
Buffalo, NY 14214
(716) 829-2056
www.buffalo.edu

New York State University—Stony Brook School of Dental Medicine
160 Rockland Hall
Stony Brook, NY 11794
(631) 632-8900
www.stonybrook.edu

New York University College of Dentistry
345 East 24th Street
New York, NY 10010
(212) 998-9800
www.nyu.edu/dental

University of North Carolina—Chapel Hill, School of Dentistry
Manning Drive and Columbia Street
Chapel Hill, NC 27599
(919) 966-1161
www.unc.edu

North Dakota State College of Science, Dental Hygiene
800 6th Street North
Wahpeton, ND 58076
(800) 342-4325
www.nodak.edu

Ohio State University School of Dentistry
305 West 12th Avenue
Columbus, OH 43210
(614) 292-2751
www.ohio-state.edu

University of Oklahoma College of Dentistry
P.O. Box 26901-DCSB 510
Oklahoma City, OK 73190
(405) 271-3530
dentistry.ouhsc.edu

Oregon Health and Science University School of Dentistry
611 SW Campus Drive
Portland, OR 97239
(503) 494-8867
www.ohsu.edu/sod

Temple University School of Dentistry
1801 North Broad Street
Philadelphia, PA 19122
(215) 204-7000
www.temple.edu/dentistry

University of Pennsylvania, Penn Dental
240 South 40th Street
Philadelphia, PA 19104-6030
(215) 898-2149
www.upenn.edu

University of Pittsburgh School of Dental Medicine
3501 Terrace Street
Pittsburgh, PA 15261
(412) 648-8880
www.dental.pitt.edu

Community College of Rhode Island, Dental Hygiene
400 East Avenue
Warwick, RI 02886
(401) 825-1000
www.ccri.edu

Medical University of South Carolina College of Dental Medicine
173 Ashley Avenue, BSB 447
P.O. Box 250507
Charleston, SC 29425
(843) 792-3811
www.musc.edu

University of South Dakota, Dental Hygiene
414 East Clark Street
Vermillion, SD 57069
(605) 677-5379
www.usd.edu/dhyg

Meharry Medical College School of Dentistry
1005 Dr. D.B. Todd, Jr. Blvd.
Nashville, TN 37208
(615) 327-6000
www.mmc.edu

University of Tennessee Health Science Center College of Dentistry
875 Union Avenue
Memphis, TN 38163
(901) 448-6200
www.utmem.edu/dentistry

Texas A&M, Baylor College of Dentistry
3302 Gaston Avenue
Dallas, TX 75246
(214) 828-8100
www.tambcd.edu

University of Texas—San Antonio Dental School
7703 Floyd Curl Drive
San Antonio, TX 78229
(210) 567-3222
www.uthscsa.edu

University of Texas Dental Branch at Houston
7000 Fannin Street
Houston, TX 77030
(713) 500-4472
www.tmc.edu

Utah Valley State College, Dental Hygiene
800 West University Parkway
Orem, UT 84058
(801) 863-INFO
www.uvsc.edu

Salt Lake Community College, Dental Hygiene
4600 South Redwood Road
Salt Lake City, UT 84123
(801) 957-4111
www.slcc.edu

Weber State University, Dental Hygiene
3850 University Circle
Ogden, UT 84408
(801) 626-6000
www.weber.edu

Vermont Technical College, Dental Hygiene
P.O. Box 500
Randolph Center, VT 05061
(800) 442-8821
www.vtc.edu

Virginia Commonwealth University School of Dentistry
520 North 12th Street, P.O. Box 980566
Richmond, VA 23298
(804) 828-9190
www.dentistry.vcu.edu

University of Washington School of Dentistry
Seattle, WA 98195
(206) 543-9198
www.dental.washington.edu

Howard University College of Dentistry
600 West Street, N.W.
Washington, DC 20059
(202) 806-0440
www.dentistry.howard.edu

West Virginia University School of Dentistry
P.O. Box 9400
Morgantown, WV 26506-9400
(304) 293-2521
www.hsc.wvu.edu

Marquette University School of Dentistry
P.O. Box 1881
Milwaukee, WI 53201-1881
(414) 288-1510
www.dental.mu.edu

INDEX

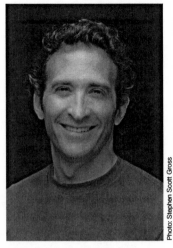

JONATHAN B. LEVINE, DMD, is a man with a mission: to give the world a reason to smile. A "smile beauty" practitioner for more than two decades, Dr. Levine is an accomplished aesthetic dentist, professor, product innovator, entrepreneur, author, and philanthropist. His dental practice, located in New York City, attracts high-profile members of the fashion community, social circuit, and Hollywood elite. In 2002, he and his wife, Stacey, co-founded the revolutionary smile beauty company GoSMILE™.

Recognized around the world as an authority on cosmetic dental procedures, Dr. Levine has always been on the cutting edge of aesthetic dentistry. He was one of the first dentists in the United States to apply porcelain veneers and among the first in the world to offer in-office tooth-whitening services. As an Associate Professor at New York University School of Dentistry and a published researcher, Dr. Levine is equally committed to influencing the next generation of dentists as he is to providing smile care and education to people in places that need it most. As such, he contributes his time and services to organizations such as Operation Smile, which works to correct childhood facial deformities around the world.

In the early 1990s, Dr. Levine developed the revolutionary GoSMILE formula for his celebrity patients who wanted to whiten their teeth simply, effectively, and safely. Soon after, GoSMILE launched at retail and its products found their way onto the selling floors of American's most prestigious specialty stores and spas.

Dr. Levine's professional affiliations include: the College of Prosthodontics, Northeast Gnathological Society, and the Academy of Osseointegration. He also sits on the Board of Medical Advisors for Klinger Advanced Aesthetics where he chairs the dental vision and initiatives for the company. A two-time All-American lacrosse player, he received his BA from Cornell University and his doctorate from the Boston University School of Dentistry, with postgraduate training in prosthodontics from New York University. Dr. Levine lives in Purchase, New York, with his wife and two sons, Cody and Julian, who bestowed GoSMILE with its name, making the company a true family affair.

CPSIA information can be obtained
at www.ICGtesting.com
Printed in the USA
FFOW04n0153020216
21055FF

9 780446 694278